It's
Twins!
Now What?

IT'S TWINS! NOW WHAT?

Vie Books is an imprint of Summersdale Publishers Ltd

Summersdale Publishers Ltd
46 West Street
Chichester
West Sussex
PO19 1RP
UK

www.summersdale.com

Printed and bound in Great Britain by CPI Group (UK) Ltd, Croydon, CR0 4YY

ISBN: 978-1-84953-812-1

Substantial discounts on bulk quantities of Summersdale books are available to corporations, professional associations and other organisations. For details contact Nicky Douglas by telephone: +44 (0) 1243 756902, fax: +44 (0) 1243 786300 or email: nicky@summersdale.com.

It's Twins!
Now What?

Tips, Advice and Real-life Experience
to Help You from Pregnancy through
to Your Babies' First Year

Jessica Bomford

Disclaimer

The material in this book is not intended as a substitute for the professional advice of a qualified therapist or healthcare professional. All children are unique, and while the book offers suggestions and recommendations to parents and other caregivers, we encourage you to use your common sense and judgement to determine when it's appropriate to seek professional advice.

Acknowledgements

Had this book been the story of my own first year of raising twins, it would have been a short one. I made precisely three entries in my diary during that period, one of which was a shopping list. Yet the seeds of this project were sown in those chaotic first twelve months, and began to take root with the encouragement and support of a wonderful group of parents with whom I congregated each week in the sanctuary of our playgroup, SE23 Twins, to discuss, commiserate and laugh, slightly hysterically, at the challenges that our twins threw at us. I feel privileged to count many of these remarkable women as my friends and am honoured that so many of them have allowed me to pass on their wise words and occasional cock-ups in this book.

In order to write *It's Twins! Now What?*, I interviewed parents of twins from across the country, many of whom I have never met, who have all allowed me to peek into their lives to extract that elusive combination of experience and humour that keeps us sane and ready to face another day. I am so grateful to every single person who has taken the time to talk to me and, in doing so, has enriched this book immeasurably.

I am also indebted to the professionals who have assisted me, some of whom have the happy coincidence of being parents of twins themselves. In particular, my thanks go to Dr Susan Bewley, whose advice and encouragement went far beyond the call of duty. Her steady voice of experience would surely calm the nerves of the most anxious expectant mother. Thank you also to Dr Bonamy Oliver, Dr Sarah Helps, Dr Saima Latif, Dr Frankie Phillips, Maggie Vaughan, Annabel Bryant and Annie Simpson, who shared their expertise so willingly.

I owe so many people so much gratitude that to pick out individuals seems somehow wrong. However, it is impossible to ignore the extra cheerleading, childcare and occasional chivvying that I received from these lovely people, so extra special thanks must go to my husband Jason Groves, and my friends Jenny Parker, Sarah Withe, Lynsey Scott, Margarita Vidiella and Sharon Street, for your invaluable support.

Final thanks go to my mum Janice, sister Lucy and my parents-in-law Sue and Rob Groves, who have helped in so many ways. I am so lucky to have you all in my life. As I write, I am thinking of my late father, Peter, who is much missed by us all, especially by his 'little chaps'.

For Jason, Kit, Alec and Harry

Contents

Chapter 1

Welcome to the Club

Everyone has a good story about the day they discovered they were having twins. It is the day your life changed, veered off at a right angle and plunged down an unmarked road. You may have punched the air with joy or dropped to the floor sobbing in shock, or perhaps you did a bit of both.

It is fair to say that in the space of a few minutes in the sonographer's room, life plans are upended, dreams reconfigured and finances shredded. Immediate practical considerations can crowd out what should be a special moment of celebration. Is our house big enough for twins? Will a double buggy fit into our car – let alone the twins themselves? Can we afford two babies? How will this affect our other children? In short: how will we cope?

If it's any consolation, every single parent who has contributed to this book has experienced this blast in the face of conflicting emotions: joy and relief at two healthy heartbeats, but understandable anxiety about what lies ahead.

The aim of this book is to equip you with the information you need to put those anxieties to rest. Think of it as your friend, someone to put an arm around your shoulders when times are tough, but who is also willing to give you the occasional home truth when required. This book is your hot-water bottle on tricky days and your gin and tonic when you need something stronger, because these pages contain hundreds of anecdotes, tips and – just as importantly – funny stories about life with twins. Not life with twins as experts imagine it to be, but real life with real twins in real families. No two stories are the same. Some advice will suit your parenting style and some won't. Some tips will be relevant for your newborn, but by the time they've hit three months you will be checking out the same chapter again for different ideas and suggestions. Babies change and our parenting style evolves, so it is useful to have as many different ideas within one book as possible.

Where medical information is required, doctors, midwives, psychiatrists and dieticians with specific expertise in twins (some of them parents of twins themselves) have shared their wisdom. However, if you have any medical concerns at all, it is important to consult your doctor or midwife immediately.

Hopefully the experiences of the many parents of twins will give you the confidence to care for your babies, and the reassurance that they were all beginners once and that no one has all the answers or always gets it right.

Sometimes, though, being forewarned can be a bit scary. Hearing about hysterical, sleep-deprived, early-hours sobbing may strike a chord of recognition once your babies are born, but as you prepare for their arrival it might be downright terrifying to imagine yourself in that position. So occasionally the brass tacks need to be covered by a bit of positive padding, and every now and then we should stop and remind ourselves of the joy that these two little people bring to our lives – and what a privilege it is to be parents of twins.

As you may have discovered already, if you thought you didn't know anyone with twins or who is a twin, you are almost certainly wrong. One of the great things about expecting or having twins is that suddenly you find everyone around you is harbouring a twin tale. A work colleague that you've known for years reveals that they are an identical twin; the supermarket checkout lady's grandchildren are twins; and suddenly Great-aunt Gussie remembers that twins do run in the family after all... she's just not sure on which side. Congratulations! You are now officially part of the worldwide twin fellowship.

> 66 We found out at the twelve-week scan and we had no idea it was twins. As the consultant was doing the scan I could see two dots and was thinking, 'Goodness, this has advanced since I had Henry (who was then five) – I can see its eyes!' Then he said, 'I've got some news...' All I could say was, 'Are they Siamese?' 99
>
> *Michelle, mum to Edward and William, four;*
> *Henry, eight; and George, ten*

> 66 After seven years of infertility we had an ICSI cycle followed, to our delight, by a positive pregnancy test. We had an early scan at six weeks at our fertility clinic and when the sonographer told us, 'Well, there are two in there,' we could not have been happier or more excited. Later, after the twins were born I came across an old diary entry which read 'planning to start fertility treatment this year, twins would be great, a boy and a girl would be ideal'. I don't think I ever really thought that we would be that lucky though... 99
>
> *Karen, mum to Millie and Alfie, three*

> 66 The sonographer declared she had something to tell us. I assumed the news was that the baby was pickled in vodka, having drunk throughout my first three months without twigging that I was in fact pregnant. So the news that there were twins was, in a tiny sense, a relief but mostly met with terror. 99
>
> *Susannah, mum to Rufus and Matilda, two*

Once news of your twin pregnancy gets out, people will either tell you that you're the luckiest people in the world or that your life is over. Commiserations mingle with congratulations. It is a confusing time, as you try to come to terms with your own reactions and deal with the responses of others.

> 66 My husband's mum had a funny nervous reaction and laughed so much she couldn't talk and had to pass the phone to his dad. He said he'd only ever seen her do that once before – at a funeral. I know that lots of people say they feel blessed by having twins, but I can honestly say I just felt terrified. The excitement I'd felt a week earlier at the prospect of having our first baby subsided into instant worry as to how we were going to cope. 99
>
> *Lynsey, mum to Ivor and George, four; and Polly, 18 months*

> 66 When I told male friends, they tended to respond in a similar way. One shook me by the hand and said, 'Congratulations, mate, you're screwed.' 99
>
> *Ming, dad to Alfred and Joseph, two*

> 66 We got really fed up with people saying how hard it was going to be for us having twins. It was the first thing everyone said. Failing IVF three times was hard. This is an absolute blast. 99
>
> *Gabby, mum to Florrie and Astrid, 12 weeks*

Meanwhile, your apparently straightforward pregnancy has rocketed up the scale to 'high risk' and suddenly all sorts of medical experts are getting involved. The reaction of your family to your news could be tempered by their concern about your health and people may start fussing over you when really all you want is reassurance – however blind – that everything will be fine and that you and your partner will make the world's best parents of twins. Try to resist the temptation to do a DIY risk-assessment on your pregnancy on the Internet. Stick to the advice you have received in hospital, which is based on you and your twins alone and, if everything is fine, simply continue to do as the experts tell you. It might be hard not to feel like a patient – after all, you are just pregnant – but try to keep life as normal as possible while you can.

For some people, the shock of a twin pregnancy is genuinely traumatic and long lasting. Many twin pregnancies are picked up at a very early stage, either because of IVF or as a result of previous complications or miscarriages. There may be medical uncertainties or the implications of such a major life change may prove overwhelming. Many people have no experience of twins at all and find the prospect of being plunged into this world daunting and isolating. For some, it is a case of saying goodbye to daydreams of a single baby and accepting the realities of coping with two – a process that does not happen overnight.

> 66 I found out very early on. I had a scan at eight weeks, where they could see two cell sacs. It was a very strange moment, with mixed emotions, as the sonographer told me the smaller foetus would probably not make it past ten weeks, as I had 'vanishing twin syndrome'. However, after a consultation with a doctor, I was told that both could develop further. Even with this reassurance, I still felt slightly confused, and not quite sure what to tell people. However, we decided to be optimistic, and christened them 'Twinkie' and 'Twinkle'. 99
>
> *Maeve, mum to Maia and Iona, four*

> ❝ As the news sank in that day, my partner became more elated while I entered a state of shock that lasted for a week or two. With a two year old already, moving from our one-bedroom flat and buying a larger car became essential. Yet this required two incomes and I would be paying my whole salary back in childcare for at least three years. No matter how I looked at it, it didn't work out. ❞
>
> *Sheena, mum to Adanna, six; and Ciara and Michael, four*

> ❝ We had never considered that we might have twins, so the discovery at the scan was a bolt from the blue. My wife said: 'My figure's going to be ruined', and I said: 'We can't afford them'. We drove home in torrential rain and when we arrived we just sat in the car in the driveway with the rain beating down for about an hour staring blankly outside, not saying anything. I thought, 'There goes the life plan.' ❞
>
> *James, dad to Rosie and Elliott, seven months; and Robin, three*

In this book, as you have seen already, parents will spare no blushes in recounting their essential survival stories about pregnancy, birth, and the first 12 months of feeding and sleeping. By reading about what other parents in your position have learnt, we hope to smooth some – sorry, it won't be all – of the bumps in the ride. throughout your first year with twins.

Because they're worth it

Twins are amazing. This may not be uppermost in your mind as you contemplate taking on a second job to buy a double buggy or listen to the unique sound of newborn babies howling in stereo.

But they are amazing. And, as parents of twins, you too are pretty special. Come on – bask in it. From now on, every parent you know, and many more that you don't, will treat you with open-mouthed respect, awe and admiration. They couldn't do it (you will hear), but you can and you are doing it!

As the powerhouses behind these two wonderful new lives, you will have semi-celebrity status bestowed upon you overnight. In pre-twin days you ambled along the pavement in obscurity, best known in the local shop for your Hobnob habit and most remembered for that New Year's Eve karaoke competition. Now you are The Twins' Parents, a legend in local parenting circles and an inspiration to all those with 'only' one baby who had previously considered themselves to be struggling. Never mind that, behind closed doors, you feel like anything but super-parents – to the outside world, you represent the pinnacle in parenting stamina.

OK, sometimes it is nice to be known by your own name and, yes, the comments can grate (more of that later), but your twins will genuinely bring joy to pretty much everyone who sees them. And when you are standing in a supermarket aisle in your slippers having gone for 24 hours without so much as a power nap or two consecutive slurps of tea, the kind comments of strangers really can lift your day. Yes, you are lucky. It had just slipped your mind.

> 66 Asking what is the best thing about having twins is like asking what your favourite song is – it's impossible not to have a top ten at the very minimum. There are so many great things about having twins and hardly any downsides, but if I had to pick one it's the magic of having two at the same time – their very 'twininess'. There have been untold joys over the past two years, from seeing your newborn twins holding hands

(although they are apparently unaware of each other) to the toddler phase with the twins' regular and exclusive giggles, and chitchat they have amongst themselves. It sounds cheesy, but most days I feel blessed to have twins, as they are to have each other in life. "

Susannah, mum to Matilda and Rufus, two

" Without a doubt having twins has been the most amazing experience of my whole life. Life is definitely harder, but much richer, too. I think the best thing is knowing that my children always have a playmate and the special shared experience of twinship. "

Karen, mum to Alfie and Millie, three

" Having twins is the best thing that has ever happened to us. It is exhausting and stressful and scary, but it is also wonderful and so special. I would never have thought such a mixed bag of emotions was possible and I wouldn't change any of it. "

Lucie, mum to Ivy and Oscar, 21 months

Fellow parents of twins will seek you out and welcome you to their exclusive club. From these people, as from this book, you will find invaluable support and understanding. Only these parents can truly understand the joys, pressures and sheer volume of nappies that caring for new twins entails.

Parenting twins gives you the unique opportunity of watching how two babies, raised in essentially the same way, at the same time, can carve out very different personalities and develop at different paces, while at the same time work as a tight team and share many similarities. You have your own nature-versus-nurture experiment right in your own sitting room. Honing your parenting skills to accommodate so many needs – plus those of other children you may have – is one of the major challenges and achievements of being a parent of twins.

66 Having twins is a great way to stop the self-blaming habit that parents can get into. Because, although we treat our twins similarly (or so we think), they have different sleeping and eating habits, and different temperaments. Tom finds it difficult to settle down to sleep; Ellie just needs a bit of rocking. In the early days, Tom consumed loads of milk, whereas for Ellie finishing a bottle was a remarkable event. Same parents, different outcomes. So it's not our fault after all! 99

Kristina, mum to Tom and Ellie, 14 months;
and George, four

66 Having had twins as our first children, although I always felt that I'd missed out on the lovely firstborn 'honeymoon' period, it made us very unfussy about them and we got good routines in place with sleep etc., which made me keep my sanity. I know lots of people with one child who had a lot less sleep in the first year than me. It definitely made me less fussy as a parent and I like that. 99

Lynsey, mum to George and Ivor, four; and Polly, 18 months

It may feel like every second person is giving birth to twins, and the figure is rising every year, but twins still account for only three per cent of the population. Twins remain a special and fascinating quirk of nature. As parents, you are allowed to be endlessly fascinated because they are your children after all. Strangers may not share your forensic interest in the colour of their poo or the fact they can 'read' a baby book at the age of three weeks, but, when the sleep clears from your eyes occasionally, you should allow yourself to stand back and appreciate what a double miracle you have created.

> " Our twins are still pretty young, but already they have adopted certain roles. Some days they are each other's best chums and then on others they are like an old married couple or a boss and employee! I love it when they wander around holding hands and muttering to each other. They really do have a special bond – I call it their 'twin bone' – which I don't think that other siblings have from such a young age. "
>
> *Jan, mum to Jamie and Sophia, two*

> " My twins, Aidan and Niamh, both call themselves Aidan. When asked their name they will both convincingly say 'Aidan', and they shout 'Aidan' to find each other or get each other's attention. I sometimes wonder if they also think they have each other's face, as obviously they don't spend much time in front of the mirror as yet (other than to occasionally kiss their own reflection). I love how from an early age they would pat each other on the back as a sign of affection, which was something as parents we used to do when burping them after a feed. "
>
> *Roisin, mum to Aidan and Niamh, 22 months*

> " Seeing the happiness they get from each other is wonderful. That bond is an unconditional friend for life, and no other relationship can be like it. To have a constant companion who understands must be truly amazing. Oh, and there's

something about two of them that multiplies the cuteness factor. 🙿

Jessica, mum to Nat and Joss, four; and Teddy, six

You may have noticed that this section is an unashamed pep talk, a big whoop whoop for twins, a reminder of some of the things that make having twins incredible. You will have your own reasons for considering it to be a privilege and a joy. It may be that, at this moment, you can't remember any of them, because there will be many times when it feels so hard to simply get through another day, never mind stop to give a cheesy thumbs up to the two tiny tyrants who are depriving you of sleep and sanity. This is why it is all the more important to give yourself a mental or actual list of some of the things that make it all worthwhile.

Bringing up twins is likely to be the hardest but most rewarding thing you will ever do. Keep telling yourself this. You are truly the jewels in the parenting crown. You have produced or are about to produce two babies who will melt your and complete strangers' hearts, give you the most wonderful double hugs and make you swell with love and pride as you watch them together.

Chapter 2

Back to Basics

Just because you are expecting twins, it doesn't mean you know much about twins or indeed have a firm grasp on how you managed to create them. Whether your twins are a genetic quirk of fate or the result of many years of fertility treatment, here's a guide to how they got here and their likely development in your womb over the next eight or nine months.

A few twin facts

About 12,500 sets of twins will be born in Britain this year, accounting for 1.5 per cent of births in this country. This is a figure that continues to rise, in part due to mothers having babies later in life, higher fertility rates and improvements in IVF (in vitro fertilisation) techniques.

Of those twins, a third will be identical and two-thirds non-identical. While there are quite a few factors that make having non-identical twins more likely for some women, identical twins present more of a mystery. There does not appear to be a genetic predisposition to having identical twins and they occur fairly consistently around the world, accounting for about 3.5 of every 1,000 births.

However, twinning rates for non-identical twins vary considerably. The highest recorded rate is among the Yoruba tribe in Nigeria, with twins accounting for 45 out of every 1,000 births, while the lowest is in Japan, with approximately six twin births out of every 1,000.

The main factors which make non-identical twins more likely are: a relatively older mother (mothers over 35 are more likely to have twins), infertility treatment, the number of previous pregnancies (the more pregnancies, the greater your chance of having twins) and a history of twins on the mother's side. Additionally, a mother of twins may be slightly taller or heavier than average, which may simply be a reflection of better nutrition.

Very rarely, twins are born with skin and internal organs fused together. Conjoined twins, sometimes called Siamese twins, occur once in every 200,000 live births.

A bit of biology

A double pregnancy occurs either when one fertilised egg (or zygote) splits into two embryos, resulting in monozygotic twins, usually known as 'identical' twins, or when two separate eggs are produced and fertilised, in which case dizygotic twins, also known as 'non-identical' or 'fraternal' twins are created.

Dizygotic twins have a placenta each. Monozygotic twins will usually share one placenta. However, if the zygote splits very early in a pregnancy, before the placenta has begun to form, some monozygotic twins can have two placentas. About a third of identical twins fall into this category, which can mean that parents are not aware that their twins are identical until they start to notice the physical similarities between their children. Some parents instigate DNA tests, which can be organised through the Multiple Births Foundation, to determine definitively what type of twins they have.

As you will see in subsequent chapters, knowing which type of twins you are carrying is essential in determining the antenatal care you require. Twins who share a placenta need the most monitoring as there is a risk of an unequal division of nutrition, causing one baby to develop more than the other. Doctors look closely at the blood flow and size of the babies for signs of twin-to-twin transfusion syndrome and intrauterine growth restriction (the latter can affect any baby). All twin pregnancies are classed as 'high risk' because of the strain an extra baby puts on the mother's body. This in turn leads to a greater likelihood of complications such as pre-eclampsia, gestational diabetes and bleeding.

Monozygotic twins share the same DNA and therefore look very alike. Although they may be 'clones' in a technical sense, they are not absolutely identical. They have very slightly different fingerprints, which is thought to be due to the foetuses touching the amniotic sac. Also, because the environment influences our DNA, certain genes will be switched off or on in different twins, meaning, for example, that both twins wouldn't necessarily suffer from conditions such as asthma or dyslexia. One might be left-handed; the other right-handed. One twin may develop a mole when the other does not, or their weights may differ. Their personalities are often very different, too. Parents-to-be of identical twins are understandably terrified of getting them muddled up but, within a few weeks, will usually start to see them as very different babies.

In contrast, dizygotic twins share half their DNA and in that respect have the same genetic relationship as with a single sibling.

The development of your twins in the womb

For the first two trimesters of your pregnancy, your twins – or rather, Twin A/1 and Twin B/2, as they will probably be called – will develop at roughly the same pace as single babies. At your first scan, the sonographer will identify each baby as either A or B and, provided the positioning of the sacs is also accurately recorded, the same twin will remain A or B until he or she is born and then gains an official name.

It is only in the last trimester that their growth slows down in comparison with a single foetus. As you might expect, you will generally feel more movement than if you were expecting one baby, usually from about 20 weeks onwards.

One piece of research suggests that the twin lying to the right in the uterus tends to be more active, while another piece casts doubt on the idea of a 'dominant' twin in the womb. You, however, may feel evidence to the contrary.

Weeks 1–6

Within 24 hours of conception, certain characteristics are already genetically predisposed in your babies, such as gender and hair colour. By the beginning of week five, the cluster of cells that makes up each baby is just about recognisable as an embryo.

Although little bigger than grains of rice and looking more like tadpoles than babies, your twins are developing quite rapidly, with primitive hearts beginning to form and starting to circulate blood, and the early development of your babies' brains, bladders, kidneys and spines under way. Although they don't work yet, their digestive systems are in place and a tube now runs from the mouth to the 'tail' of each embryo, from which the stomach, liver, pancreas and bowels will develop. Everything is covered by a thin layer of see-through skin.

Weeks 6–12

During this period, some facial features – such as the eyes, nose, ears and mouth – become recognisable and the shapes of your babies change. Their heads grow rapidly in this period to accommodate an ever-expanding brain. By week eight, the middle ear, responsible for both balance and hearing, is formed. Tooth buds for milk teeth are in place within the forming jawbones. Elsewhere, your babies' arms are lengthening, webbed hands now develop separate fingers and by week ten touch pads have developed on the end of the fingertips. Most muscles are in place, which can be seen as jerky movements on your ultrasound scans. Also, by week ten, your babies' hearts will have developed into four chambers and will be beating at twice your own heart rate. This will slow and continue to do so as the two babies become more mature.

Weeks 12–16

Your twins will be losing their 'question mark' shapes now, and filling out into more recognisable 'baby' forms. They have also graduated to a new technical term and move from embryo to foetus status. During this period, each baby's weight will increase from just over half an ounce to just over four, so it is a period of rapid growth.

Their heads continue to appear relatively large, but the rest of their bodies are starting to catch up. The eyes are now positioned at the front of the face with the eyelids closed, and taste buds have formed. Genitalia are becoming increasingly obvious, with a rudimentary penis visible on male foetuses. Also during this period, the liver begins to function, as do the kidneys, and by the 16th week water in their stomachs and urine in their bladders may be detected via ultrasound. They are swallowing amniotic fluid and then expelling it through urination.

There is more movement going on, too, though it is unlikely to be strong enough to be felt yet. Research conducted by Umberto Castiello of the University of Padova, which studied video footage of twins in utero at 14 weeks, found that, although separated by a thin membrane, the twins touched each other head to head, arm to arm, and head to arm. Researchers concluded that these were not reflexes, but planned movements.

Weeks 16–20

By the end of this period, you may well have felt the first few kicks from your twins, who will each be about 18 cm long. Some mums say they can distinguish between the two; others aren't so sure. During this stage, your babies' lower halves are rapidly catching up with their top halves and their bodies will appear more in proportion as a result. Inside the ovaries of a baby girl are the eggs she will be born with.

Weeks 20–24

Your twins' skin pigment is now starting to form, it is no longer translucent as fat is starting to be laid down under the skin, which will help them maintain their proper body temperatures. The surface of their skin has a fine layer of hair and a thick coating of white vernix, a waxy layer that protects the babies from their long submersion in amniotic fluid. Your babies' nervous and skeletal systems are continuing to mature, resulting in more sophisticated movements, including somersaults and kicks. The babies' hearing has improved and it is thought that they can recognise your voice now.

They have started to form a pattern of sleeping and waking. Research shows that twins are remarkably synchronised on this front, and in 94 per cent of cases are likely to be asleep or awake at the same time – alas, that synchronicity does not always extend to the mum, too.

The 24-week stage marks the beginning of the 'viability' of your babies – the point where they could, with considerable medical intervention, survive outside the womb. By 24 weeks they will weigh approximately 1 lb 7 oz each.

Weeks 24–28

It is around this point that your twins' growth slows down compared with single babies, probably due to lack of space. During this period, your babies' eyelids will open, hair continues to grow, facial features become more defined and the major organs continue to mature. By the end of this stage, your twins could weigh about 2 lb 7 oz each.

Weeks 28–32

This is a period of rapid brain development and continued growth. Your babies will put on approximately another 1 lb 2 oz each as they accrue more fat. All the organs are in working order with the exception of the lungs. Meanwhile, the babies' taste buds can already allow them to differentiate between sweet and bitter flavours, and their mouths open and close regularly. At 28 weeks, your babies have a functioning sense of smell, which is not impeded by amniotic fluid.

Weeks 32–36

Your babies' lungs will now start to mature in readiness for taking their first breath. Your twins continue to put on weight, but at a slower rate than a single baby at the same stage. Space is very cramped now – they may be almost as uncomfortable as you. By 36 weeks, your babies may weigh about 4 lb 14 oz each.

Weeks 36–40

The majority of twin pregnancies end by or during week 38. Due to some evidence of a slightly increased risk of foetal death beyond 38 weeks, induction is usually offered after this point. Hardly any twin pregnancies will be overdue. From the point of view of development, your babies are fully formed and as ready for birth as they will ever be.

Chapter 3

Stuff and Nonsense

Farewell, then, to minimalist living and hello to life in the shadow of a heap of baby-related paraphernalia. Now is the time to start the lengthy process of establishing what stuff is essential, desirable or an expensive waste of floor space. The good news is that you don't need as much as you think you do – alas, this is probably still more than will fit comfortably into your house.

Equipping yourself for the arrival of your twins, particularly if they are your first children, is a really exciting process but, unless your home is of palatial proportions and you have a similarly expansive bank balance, try not to get carried away with the matching cuteness of it all. There may be some stonking investments to be made – such as a new car or even house – which could knock quite a hole in your budget.

So, rein in the monogrammed cots and life-sized cuddly giraffes for the time being. Start with the basics and add stuff when you need it. Some parents don't like the idea of buying second-hand gear for their newborns, but if you are a bargain hunter there is a lot of equipment in great nick out there (often via twins club forums or nearly-new sales) which will save you heaps of cash.

You will find an ever-increasing range of twin-specific gadgets, carriers and equipment on the market, some of which may be really useful. However, just because someone has invented a thingy which allows you to carry both twins on your back whilst simultaneously vacuuming, tap-dancing and expressing milk, that doesn't mean you have to use it – or feel guilty about not using it.

Tucking up the babies in a pram and putting your feet up in the traditional way is a pretty good option, too.

The buggy

Double buggies are becoming ever more manoeuvrable and manageable, and a good range is now stocked by the majority of mainstream pushchair suppliers. For the most part, their prices are still stratospheric, but your buggy will be your constant companion for the next three years and, if you get the right one, this should be money well spent.

Issues to consider when choosing your buggy:

► How big is the boot of your car and will the buggy fit into it?

► Can you lift the buggy into your car boot?

► Will you be using public transport? If so, the buggy needs to be super-manoeuvrable and not too heavy

► Will it fit through your front door?

► How easy is it to push and steer, preferably with one hand?

► Where will you put the buggy at home? Is a collapsible buggy practical?

► Is there enough space underneath the seats to stash your shopping and the changing gear while you are out and about?

► Can your newborns lie flat or is there a pram/carry-cot option for when they are tiny?

► Will your buggy grow with your children? If it's a buggy to which you can attach car seats for newborns, how will it perform when your twins are toddlers?

The best place to road test many different types of double buggies in one hit is at a meeting of your local twins club. Most parents are more than happy for you to wheel their buggies about and be quizzed on their merits. A quick trip one morning could save you hours of research.

> 66 My double buggy was probably my best piece of equipment – it was very expensive but excellent. We walked for miles with it and it saved me from total madness! Essentially, I wanted one with carry cots that would fit through my front door, that I could put the car seats on (which I did a lot!) and that I could run with. 99
>
> *Lindsay, mum to Serafina and Alex, 22 months*

Car seats

You may buy a car seat as part of your buggy 'travel system', but if not, first car seats are rear-facing and are secured using an adult seat belt or ISOFIX. The joy of these seats is that they are portable and have a handle, so they allow you to lift your sleeping babies in and out of the car without disturbing them. Make sure you get some guidance on fitting the seats; many stores offer a free fitting service. Don't leave it until the hospital car park to familiarise yourself with the manual's fine print.

Slings

Slings can be really useful, particularly if one twin is very grisly and unsettled. They enable you to be mobile while soothing the baby at the same time. There are now a variety of slings that can accommodate two babies – either one at the front and one at the back or two (small) babies at the front. However, carrying two babies around for any length of time can get pretty tiring, and the human packhorse approach is not for everyone. Make sure you follow the instructions carefully to ensure the babies are safely strapped in and that you are not putting too much strain on your back.

Clothes

There are so many adorable baby clothes around that you would have to be made of stone not to splash out on at least a few cute matching outfits before your little ones arrive. However, once they do, your twins are most likely to spend their first few months dressed almost exclusively in Babygros with a vest underneath. Bear in mind that babies get through a lot of outfits each day due to leaking nappies, dribbling, milk stains and sick. Babygros are easy to get on and off, and are straightforward to wash. Some Babygros are like a long dress that poppers up along the bottom and these are even easier to use.

Avoid buying too many clothes in advance. The 'newborn' size might seem tiny in the shop but may well swamp your twins, especially if they come early. You are more likely to need 'tiny baby' or even 'premature baby', but you can't count on this, so just buy the minimum until you know exactly what you need. Once they have arrived, you will need, as a rough guide, about three vests and Babygros per baby per day.

Monitors

There is a baby monitor out there to suit any budget and level of parental anxiety. Everyone will have their own views on whether they require the light shows, night vision, lullabies and temperature alerts – and will choose accordingly. Monitors also give you the option of enlivening dull visits by broadcasting your whispered comments directly to your guests in the lounge – in digital quality.

Bear in mind that, while monitors can be great for allowing you to get on while the babies are napping, excessive listening-in can mean that you are straining to hear your little ones breathing instead of getting on with the important business of having a rest yourself. It is usually possible to hear a baby crying from most rooms in most average-sized houses without the aid of digital technology. It is even more possible to hear two.

Sleeping arrangements

Many parents of twins find that it works extremely well to have their twins sharing a cot at first. You must position the babies so that their feet are safely pointing towards 'their' own end of the cot, lying with their heads in the centre of the cot. Tuck covers securely under their arms so they cannot slip over their heads. Make sure the mattress is well fitting, firm, flat, clean and waterproof, and cover it with a fitted sheet. Initially, Moses baskets may seem cosier, particularly if the babies are small, and you may prefer this option if you have the space, but they are not essential. Again, make sure the babies are positioned safely with their feet at the end of the basket. You can also buy cots that attach directly to the side of your bed, which can make night-time feeds a lot easier.

Think about where your cot or cots will go. Make sure it is away from radiators and any blind cords, which will be a safety hazard once the babies can stand in their cots. Your babies will not need excessive heat during the night, about 18°C is ideal.

Twins who sleep in the same room or share a cot can, of course, wake each other up, but they are so used to each other's presence that they are likely to sleep through disturbances.

You will need at least four fitted sheets with your cots (again, there are lots of leakages) as well as four cellular blankets (which are light with little holes in them and help to keep the babies' temperatures regular) and cotton cot sheets.

When the babies clear 8 lb 8 oz, they can wear Grobags, a handy sleeping bag that attaches over their shoulders with poppers. A Grobag saves a whole load of faffing around with little blankets and sheets – you can be pretty confident your baby is the right temperature and you know they're not going to wriggle out of it.

> 66 Friends who had twins gave us a great tip to put a muslin cloth under their heads (and tuck it round the mattress) so that if the babies dribbled on it (one did, one didn't) you only needed to change the muslin and not the whole sheet. 99
>
> **Jo, mum to Iris and Dexter, two**

Some parents find a travel cot useful if they are attempting to split the feeding load at night and want to give one partner a complete break by moving the whole feeding and sleeping operation to a different room. Later, the cot comes into its own again as a safe place to put newly crawling babies when you need to go to the toilet or make a cup of tea. In between times, it is relatively easy to store.

Nappies and changing stations

Don't overstock with nappies until you know what size your babies are – the last thing you want is an industrial quantity of a size that takes them months to grow into.

As a rough guide, you will need ten nappies per day per baby. Keep a regular check on supermarkets for their two-for-one offers on nappies.

With two babies to attend to, a lot of parents set up changing stations upstairs and downstairs, or in two different rooms, for convenience. These can be as simple as a changing mat on the floor or a dedicated changing unit, depending on your budget and space. If you have had a C-section, you will find a changing table very helpful as you won't have to bend over too much. A changing mat on the floor can be hard on your back.

Feeding kit

For obvious reasons, you will need more 'kit' for bottle-feeding than breastfeeding, but whatever you are planning on the feeding front, it won't be long before muslin squares are your fashion accessories of choice. You will usually have at least two draped over you and another few dotted over the sofa for coordination purposes. They are useful for mopping up pretty much anything and dry very quickly, so are an essential piece of kit.

If you are considering breastfeeding, think about where you are likely to be feeding your babies – for example, on the sofa or a big armchair – and try to visualise yourself with the twins. Some breastfeeding chairs, designed for women with one baby, are not big enough to accommodate a feeding cushion, so bear this in mind if you are going to invest in new 'feeding' furniture.

A twin-specific feeding cushion (one on which you can feed both babies at the same time) comes very highly recommended by many mums of twins. These cushions often fasten around the mum and provide a useful 'platform' for breastfeeding. Other women prefer a pile of more conventional cushions, but this tends to be improvised once the twins arrive. Investing in supportive equipment that is going to keep your twins securely in place and protect your back is important. The improvised version is all very well, but making sure your babies are in a safe and comfortable position to feed should be your starting point.

A lot of expectant mums invest in an electric double breast pump to speed up expressing milk. These can be expensive and many women struggle to express as well as feed two babies – but don't find that out until they start feeding. For this reason, you can often get virtually unused breast pumps second hand. It is also possible to hire them from either the pump manufacturer or a number of baby product retailers.

> 66 I had a hands-free double breast pump which you wore like a bra. It sounds ridiculous, but it took me ages to express, so with this I could do the hoovering while I pumped. It probably saved me hours! 99
>
> *Shelley, mum to Iris and Amelia-Rose, 18 months*

If you are likely to bottle-feed, opinion varies on the number of bottles you will need, and there are a lot of different sizes and teats, but start with about eight to ten small bottles. You will also need a microwave or electric steriliser. Most parents recommend an extra kettle purely for bottles and some suggest a flask for instant night-time feeding water.

Depending on your budget, you may not need to bother with all that as the miracle of modern science brings you bottle-making machines, which whip up a bottle of formula in a couple of minutes.

You may also need to rearrange things in the kitchen to make way for your imminent feeding station. Having an area where you can keep your feeding equipment clean and separate will help you to stay organised and ensure you are not left without a clean bottle – whenever it is demanded. In the early days, some parents keep a small whiteboard or a notepad nearby so that they can record each feed and the amount consumed by each baby.

See Chapter 10 for further advice on feeding.

---

66 My best bits of equipment were 'self-feeding' bottles. When the girls were only a few months old I could prop them up on the sofa and they could feed by themselves – it's a bit like sucking a dummy. I also found they needed less burping because they were so upright when they were drinking. 99

Myfanwy, mum to Rojin and Narin, six; and Shivan, nine

66 A friend gave me two bouncy chairs, which she'd used for her twins. I can honestly say the day she dropped them round was the moment I actually started coping! The girls were about eight weeks. I could suddenly feed them both at the same time, propped up safely and at the perfect angle, and when I had to wind one I could rock the other with a minute movement of one foot. The girls loved those chairs – they used them till they were two and soon got used to rocking themselves. They progressed through bottles I was holding, through to bottles they were holding, through to early weaning foods in those chairs. I recommend them to all new mums now, but especially for twins. 99

Helen, mum to Sophia and Hannah, three

Bath-time kit

Opinion differs as to whether it is necessary to invest in a specific baby bath. It is perfectly possible to bath new babies in an average-sized bath, but a baby bath can make the process feel a bit more manageable, is cosier for your babies and uses less water. You can buy bath thermometers, but your elbow is a cheaper and just as effective option.

There are various bath chairs on the market, such as a towelling 'slope', which sits in the bath and allows you to lay your baby on it so it is properly supported, while giving you the peace of mind that he or she is not about to slip out of your hands. For safety reasons, do not try to bath your babies at the same time. As they get older and stronger you may feel confident in doing this, but when they are newborn only bath one at a time.

Many parents recommend investing in a couple of baby bath towels with built-in hoods, which keep your twins nice and cosy while they wait for their turn in the water.

Digital thermometer

There will be numerous times in the coming years when you need to check your children's temperatures, so invest in something reliable and accurate. A digital thermometer, which works when placed under your baby's armpit, is more reliable for small babies than one that takes the temperature from their ear.

Entertainment items

Newborn babies don't do an awful lot, except sleep (if you're lucky) and drink, but you will probably still find that after a while your lounge is arranged into a carousel of short-term entertainment stations to give a little variety to their waking hours and – just as importantly – your day.

Fortunately, newborn babies find most things – particularly movement – fascinating so it is not necessary to invest in much official entertainment.

Having said that, here are some entertainment options:

- **A play gym** with toys dangling down for the babies to gaze at and, as they get older, grab and chew. You can clip different toys overhead if you want to vary the view. Both babies will fit on one standard mat when they are newborn.

- **A swinging chair** – Some parents of twins swear by these as the next best thing to an extra pair of hands. It swings automatically, plays music and often has something dangly for the baby to look at. The downsides are that they take up quite a lot of room – and some babies hate them.

- **Black-and-white board books** – Newborns have quite blurry eyesight and babies will not have full-colour vision until they are about five months old, but your twins can be entertained by the bold black-and-white patterns in these books.

66 We created three places for play, two mats and a sit-up inflatable ring or a door bouncer. This way you can move them around to other areas of interest, especially as the months roll on. Vary the toys you get out each day and introduce them gradually throughout the day. We made three boxes, one was 'tactile', i.e. contained materials to feel such as silky, furry, cotton, cardboard and plastic; one was for hard investigative toys; and one was for soft toys such as teddy bears etc. I tended to rotate which ones I gave them. Materials such as sarongs are great for shaking over your babies, they love it and the brighter the patterns the better. I used to do this to music whilst they sat in their chairs. 99

Kaz, mum to Nathaniel and Reuben, five

Other stuff

If budget, imagination and house size were no limit, it would be possible to buy pretty much any gadget for any task you are likely to face in the coming year. Our own space constraints in this book mean that there's no room for recommendations on designer changing bags, baby butt fans (yes, really), packs of 'chic' disposable morning-sickness barf bags or other items of kit that you may view as essential. However, rest assured that there's plenty more where they came from. Hurry, while stocks last.

Chapter 4

Pregnancy

Let's face it: women carrying twins pack a lot into their pregnancies. Not only do you manage to produce two babies in less time than many women take to create one, but in doing so you defy gravity with a bump of such enormity that it is destined to be discussed by friends and strangers alike for years to come.

As your babies are growing at about the same rate as single babies for at least two-thirds of the pregnancy, space is clearly at a premium and, as far as your tummy is concerned, the only way is out.

Many women report that by about 30 weeks they feel as big as they imagined they would be at full term, which is well worth considering when you are planning your work schedule, maternity leave and exercise regime.

As a high-risk pregnancy, you will be attending a lot of appointments with midwives, consultants and sonographers – and if you are carrying identical twins, this monitoring will be increased yet further. You'll have scan pictures lining your hamster cage by the time your twins arrive as well as the ability to produce a urine sample in 30 seconds flat at any time of the night or day.

Lots of women find it reassuring to know that both their health and their babies' progress is being looked after so diligently, but it can be difficult having to take lots of time off work for appointments or having to juggle your other children in order to attend yet another scan. Don't be tempted to skip appointments – as you will see later in this chapter, certain conditions such as pre-eclampsia and twin-to-twin transfusion syndrome are potentially fatal and are usually picked up by medical staff before you would notice a single symptom.

It is worth reiterating that if you are concerned about anything at all during your pregnancy, see your doctor or midwife immediately. Trust your instincts and get any niggling worries checked out. Given the fact that half of women pregnant with twins will give birth prematurely, it is also important that you are familiar with the signs of preterm labour, which you'll find listed on p.95.

Being pregnant

Fortunately, double the joy doesn't necessarily mean double the morning sickness. As with any pregnancy, the symptoms vary enormously. Some women do not experience nausea and sickness at all, while others are floored by it almost from the start.

Equally, some women will develop strange food preferences and a heightened sense of smell or taste, while others won't. However, while the vagaries of symptoms are different for any pregnant woman, there are certain issues that all women expecting twins will face.

Common issues experienced during pregnancy:

▶ You will feel more tired, particularly from the middle of the second trimester at 20 weeks. For some this is manageable; for others extra naps need to be built into the day, which is not straightforward for anyone, particularly if you are at work or looking after other children.

▶ You are carrying two babies, which often means two placentas and always means more amniotic fluid, so you will be bigger. You are likely to look pregnant earlier. By about 30 weeks, you will be feeling pretty heavy and, in come cases, sluggish.

▶ You will need to eat more to sustain yourself and therefore your two babies. Carry snacks around with you to keep your energy levels up during the day.

66 In the first 12 weeks I wondered why I didn't have extra strong pregnancy symptoms given I had two babies in me. I worried because I wasn't sick, wasn't that nauseous and only a little bit more tired. The main things I had were breathlessness and a really bunged up nose that was and still is very snotty each morning. 99

Lisa, 22 weeks pregnant

66 I developed an almost super-human sense of smell. In fact, that's how I first knew I was pregnant – I was at work and my colleague came through the door and when she spoke I could smell her breath! At that moment, I just knew. 99

Gabby, mum to Astrid and Florrie, 12 weeks

Common complaints

Indigestion and heartburn

A combination of hormonal changes and your growing womb pressing on your stomach makes indigestion a very common problem in twin pregnancies. Heartburn, a burning pain in the chest caused by stomach acid passing from your stomach into your oesophagus, can also be extremely unpleasant.

To avoid these complaints, try eating little and often, and make some dietary changes to cut out chocolate, cheese, spicy foods and tomatoes. Failing that, see your GP as there is medication that can help these conditions – but check the medications' labels carefully as usually they should not be taken at the same time as iron supplements.

Anaemia

If you are feeling tired, looking pale or feeling faint, you may be anaemic. Anaemia is a condition that occurs when you don't have enough haemoglobin in your blood or have fewer red blood cells than normal. Red blood cells contain haemoglobin, a red pigment that gives blood its colour. The job of haemoglobin is to carry oxygen around the body so when red blood cells and therefore haemoglobin is low the blood fails to give the body's tissues sufficient amounts of oxygen.

See your GP, who may recommend iron supplements, and check the advice later in this chapter for tips on how to incorporate more iron-rich foods into your diet.

Nasal complaints

Your blood flow increases dramatically in pregnancy and an unexpected side effect of this can be that the mucus membranes in your nose have a greater blood supply, leading to a runny nose or bunged-up feeling.

Bleeding gums

Increased blood supply can also be blamed for an increased likelihood of bleeding gums during pregnancy.

Backache

With considerably more weight to support, it is not surprising that backache is an extremely common problem. The ligaments in your body are becoming softer and will stretch to prepare you for labour, which can put extra strain on the joints of your lower back and pelvis. Any sort of heavy lifting should be avoided during your pregnancy. You should try to work at surfaces high enough to prevent any stooping as well as sit on supportive chairs. See your doctor for help if the pain becomes severe or persistent.

Lack of sleep

As the pregnancy progresses, this becomes a major issue for most women. It becomes very hard to get comfortable or to stay comfortable for any length of time. Sleeplessness is related to central brain activity and alertness, so some experts argue that this happens to pregnant women as a way to prepare them for listening out for the babies once born. Not much comfort when you are lying awake at 3 a.m.

Experiment with different sleeping positions, such as using pillows to sleep sitting up or put a cushion behind your back or between your legs. You could also try the recovery position (lying on your side with one knee raised above the other). Take naps during the day, if possible, to top up on sleep.

Acne

You are about to embark on a defining experience of womanhood, yet suddenly your skin has gone back to its pesky 13-year-old self. Getting acne during pregnancy is a result of the sudden surge of hormones through your body and changes to your immune system. Spots usually depart once the babies arrive.

Carpal tunnel syndrome

This is a tingling sensation, numbness and sometimes pain in the hand and fingers, which tends to develop gradually. The thumb, index finger and middle finger are most commonly affected. The syndrome is caused by the pressing down of one of the nerves that controls sensation and movement in your hands. There are various treatments available, including wearing a wrist splint or having a steroid injection. Failing this, surgery may be recommended.

> ❝ I feel like I've had every symptom/problem possible. Sickness, spots, headaches, sciatica (in both legs), back pain, indigestion and acid reflux, not to mention stuffing my face! Plus now that I'm getting bigger, walking and even standing for longer periods of time are proving near impossible. I'm just feeling very heavy and unable to get on with my normal life at the moment, sleeping is also a nightmare as my legs tend to go a bit numb as I'm trying to get to sleep and just finding a comfortable position is so difficult. ❞
>
> *Rosie, 30 weeks pregnant with twin girls,*
> *and mum to Theo, eight*

More serious complications

Pre-eclampsia

This condition can affect women without them even knowing it and is usually picked up by high blood pressure readings and protein in the urine. Other indicators can be severe headaches, and sudden swelling or puffiness of ankles and hands. If signs of pre-eclampsia are present, you will be kept under close observation, sometimes in hospital. If undetected, this condition can threaten both the babies and the mother.

> ❝ I went into hospital for a routine check-up with the midwife at 33 weeks and never left. She found protein in my urine so I had to stay in for a 24-hour urine check. I was certain I'd be going home after that because I felt absolutely fine, but after getting the results I was told I would be staying in until my twins were

born. After a week my blood pressure started rising and the
boys were induced at 34 weeks and five days. **)**

Jo, mum to Iris and Dexter, two

Gestational diabetes

Some women develop such high blood sugar levels during pregnancy
that their bodies are unable to make enough insulin to absorb it all.
You may feel very hungry or thirsty and need to urinate a lot. Once
detected, this can be controlled with a change in diet, monitoring
and sometimes insulin.

Vaginal bleeding

Although very worrying, this is quite common. The Twins and
Multiple Births Association found that one in four women expecting
twins reported some vaginal bleeding during pregnancy. It does not
necessarily mean there is a problem with one or both of the babies,
but it is essential that you tell your doctor straight away so that any
more serious complications can be ruled out.

Intrauterine growth restriction

Sometimes scans will reveal that one twin is not getting enough
sustenance from the placenta and that its growth is affected. If this
happens, you will be monitored very closely, but doctors will leave
the babies in utero for as long as possible unless the twin is at risk.
Unlike twin-to-twin transfusion syndrome, it is unlikely that there
will be a sudden deterioration in the condition of the smaller twin,
and parents can feel reassured that regular scans will pick up any
changes that are likely to put the smaller twin at risk. Most IGR
babies compensate for their lack of sustenance for a long time –

as adults would if we went on a diet – before the effects become dangerous. This does not stop it being frightening and stressful for the parents, who need to prepare for the likelihood of a premature birth as well as coping with the additional risks to their baby.

66 Scans had picked up at 20 weeks that there was a problem with intrauterine growth restriction so we were monitored really closely. One week our normal consultant was away and we had somebody else who started telling us that we would have to start thinking about letting one twin die to 'save' the other one. We were really scared. Then our consultant came back and said we were nowhere near the stage of having to think like that. He was brilliant and so experienced, but I made a complaint against the other consultant and requested that she was not involved in our care again. 99

Yasmeen, mum to Khalil and Eesa, three; and Hanifah, 11

Twin-to-twin transfusion syndrome

This is a very alarming condition that affects 10–15 per cent of twins who share a placenta. In normal circumstances, your placenta contains blood vessels that allow the blood to flow evenly between your twins. However, twin-to-twin transfusion syndrome (TTTS) arises when these blood vessels distribute blood unequally to the babies, causing problems to both the twin that is not getting enough, referred to as the 'donor', and the twin who is receiving too much, the 'recipient'. The donor twin becomes smaller and is surrounded by very little amniotic fluid, while the recipient twin is put under strain by having too much blood, which it compensates for by producing too much amniotic fluid.

This condition can develop at any time, but is most commonly detected before 24 weeks. It can happen to anyone and is not caused by your actions.

Symptoms that can indicate TTTS include:

▶ Breathlessness

▶ Sudden, noticeable weight gain over a short period of time

▶ Increased thirst

▶ A shiny looking, tight or uncomfortable tummy

If you have any suspicion that you are suffering from TTTS, you must see your consultant urgently. If TTTS is diagnosed, you will be very closely monitored. Sometimes doctors will suggest laser ablation therapy to separate the blood vessels in the placenta.

It is difficult to overstate the stress and fear experienced by parents whose twins are diagnosed with TTTS. It is a condition that changes very rapidly, is entirely outside your control and puts your twins at great risk. Trying to keep negative thoughts at bay and focusing on the present is something that everyone facing TTTS struggles with. There are a number of excellent support groups for parents in the same situation and many people find it very reassuring to be in touch with others who understand how they feel. See the Resources and Further Reading section for full details.

66 A scan at 18 weeks confirmed TTTS and laser surgery was recommended. We were so frightened – the statistics seemed to be against the babies. We'd not yet met them and we might

lose them – it was horrifying. The hardest thing was thinking about losing one. The fact that they were identical twins and you would always know he was a twin.

I was awake during laser surgery as I'd had a spinal epidural. I had an incision near my belly button and a camera and laser were inserted. At the end of the procedure they turned the screen round and we could see George. I've actually got the DVD of the whole thing, it took me about six months to watch it, but you can see their faces. It's something not many people can have (or would want to go through), but it is special for them now.

I felt lighter – they took out 2.5 litres of fluid and my bump wasn't so high. I was a lot more comfortable.

You have to wait three and a half hours after the surgery for a viability scan. It was a frightening time – we just sat there, not saying much, just waiting. All I wanted to hear was that there were two heartbeats. I remember looking up at the ceiling, not at the screen, until I heard they'd found both heartbeats. 〞

Alyson, mum to George and Archie, eight months; and Erin, 12

〝 At 19 weeks I was told there was twin-to-twin transfusion syndrome – Riley had almost no fluid – or was 'shrink-wrapped', as I called it – and Henley was drowning in it. It was a really frightening time because the doctors made it clear that they thought we'd only end up with one baby, or maybe none. Every time I went for a scan I didn't know if there would be two heartbeats. It sounds awful, but my husband and I went through every 'what if' and went over every possible outcome because that was the only way we could cope with it.

At 29 weeks I went for a routine scan and the nurse told me: 'We need to go to theatre and get the babies out now.'

> Although it was frightening, I also felt a sense of relief – I felt that I couldn't help them when they were inside but now, even though there were lots of risks, we could do something for them. 〝
>
> *Clare, mum to Henley and Riley, 19 months; Lexi, three; and Kaysie, nine*

Vanishing twin syndrome (VTS)

Sometimes an early scan can show two foetal heartbeats and two foetal sacs, but by the 12-week scan one may have disappeared. This is because one of the embryos failed to thrive and has been reabsorbed into the womb. This is referred to as vanishing twin syndrome and is thought to have no physical effect on the surviving baby, although it is, of course, extremely distressing to experience as parents.

Preterm labour

For advice on recognising the signs of preterm labour, see Chapter 7.

Nutrition

With all the monitoring and hospital visits, it is easy to feel more like a patient than someone who just happens to be pregnant with more than one baby. For this reason, try to maintain your normal routine as much as possible for as long as possible – unless you are a weightlifter or a trapeze artist.

Women pregnant with twins are, of course, advised to eat healthily and yet the advice given (if any is provided at all) is vague, based on very little twin-specific research and often leaves mothers-to-be clueless about how much they should be eating. The NHS promotes a Healthy Start supplement for pregnant women (it is the same whether women are expecting one or two babies), which contains folic acid, vitamin C and vitamin D. Current NHS guidelines suggest that women pregnant with twins have their iron levels checked at 20 weeks and 28 weeks, and supplements may be recommended.

There are very few twin-specific recommendations from professional nutritional organisations in the UK, so this book draws on American research as a guide. This information should be used in conjunction with advice you receive from your doctor or medical advisers. If you suffer from gestational diabetes or any other specific condition, it is important you follow dietary advice from your doctor. Do not take vitamin supplements without consulting your doctor as too many vitamins can be damaging or have side effects. The best way of ensuring that you have the right nutrients is to incorporate them into your diet.

The NHS guidance for women expecting twins is exactly the same as that for any pregnant woman, regardless of the fact that you are carrying two babies. There is also no advice about how much weight is sensible and necessary to gain during the course of your pregnancy. In the absence of official twin-tailored advice, it is a case of listening to your body and trying to fill it healthily over the course of a day with three regular meals and two to three snacks. You may dread piling on weight that could be difficult to shift once the babies are born, but your body is giving life to two little people and needs a healthy, energy-giving diet in order to sustain everyone.

❝ In pregnancy the body becomes much more efficient and adapts to the extra demands of the babies. There is a metabolic change and a greater ability to absorb nutrients. Look at your normal diet and try to tweak it to include healthier foods. Don't skip meals – that's crucial – and always have a healthy snack to hand so that you don't have to resort to a chocolate bar or crisps when you get hungry.

In the third trimester women carrying twins often can't eat big meals as they haven't got much space left! So small, nutrient-dense snacks at this time are really important. You need a good boost of nutrients without excessive sugar and fats.

My recommendation is always to go for food sources rather than supplements because what you get from the whole food matrix is far more than you get from taking a pill. If you're eating a chilli or Bolognese sauce, you're not just getting iron from the meat, you're getting zinc, vitamin B12, protein, some healthy fats, extra fibre, and extra vitamins and minerals. If you just have the supplement you're getting the nutrients but you're not getting the whole package. 》

Dr Frankie Phillips, dietician, and mum to Sian and Natalie, seven

Let's be clear about how clever your body is being as your babies grow and develop. Your blood volume will have increased by 50–70 per cent by 20 weeks. You will have a greater placenta mass, which results in a big increase in steroid and hormone production. These hormonal changes drive a big surge in carbohydrate demand. As you have seen in Chapter 2, your babies are developing at a very rapid rate, and to do so they are using your bodily stocks of vitamins and nutrients.

American doctors William Goodnight and Roger Newman describe a multiple gestation as a state of 'accelerated starvation', whereby the mother's body is being starved in order to sustain her two passengers. Goodnight and Newman recommend a diet made up of 20 per cent protein, such as lean meat, fish, skin-free poultry, eggs, pulses, peas, tofu, cottage cheese, milk and cheese; 40 per cent low glycaemic index (GI) carbohydrates, such as brown rice, wholewheat/multigrain bread and pasta, boiled potatoes, green vegetables, beans and lentils; and 40 per cent fats, such as nuts, seeds, oily fish (no more than two portions a week) and avocado. (See the Resources and Further Reading section at the end of the book for how to access Goodnight and Newman's research.)

It can be a bit daunting to think about overhauling your diet as well as everything else you are juggling at the moment, but each essential vitamin and nutrient in the list below is helping your babies to develop and grow, as well as keeping *you* strong and healthy.

Small changes can make a big difference, so any tweak you can make to your food – such as swapping crisps for a snack of crunchy carrots and hummus, or adding vegetables to a dish – will instantly make it healthier.

Calcium

Your babies need calcium to build strong bones and teeth, but it is also essential for healthy hearts, nerves and muscles. Your babies draw their calcium from what you eat, but if that is not sufficient they will extract it from your bone mass. Research shows that most women do not consume nearly enough calcium in pregnancy. Bear in mind that only about a third of the calcium you ingest will actually be absorbed into your body.

Good sources of calcium are: milk, dairy products, tofu, fortified soya milk, yoghurts and puddings, fortified rice/oat drinks, broccoli, white bread, sesame seeds, tahini, nuts, and dried fruit such as apricots and figs.

Vitamin D

This is necessary to regulate the levels of calcium and phosphates in your body – these keep bones and teeth healthy. Deficiencies can cause weak teeth and bones and, in rare cases, rickets. We get vitamin D from the sun so women subjected to bed rest in pregnancy are particularly vulnerable to deficiency.

Good sources of vitamin D are: most margarines, fortified brands of soya milk, yoghurts and desserts (check the label), fortified breakfast cereals, eggs and dried skimmed milk.

Folic acid

Folic acid can help to prevent birth defects known as 'neural tube defects', including spina bifida, which is when a fault in the development of the spinal cord and surrounding bones leaves a gap or split in the spine. Folic acid should be taken very early in pregnancy, ideally from when you are trying to conceive until you are 12 weeks pregnant.

There are foods that contain folate (the natural form of folic acid), such as green leafy vegetables and brown rice. Some breakfast cereals and fat spreads, such as margarine, have folic acid added to them. However, it is hard to get enough folate from food alone, which is why supplements are recommended for all pregnancies. There is no specific NHS recommendation for women pregnant with twins to take any more than the standard daily dose of 400 micrograms.

Iron

See Anaemia (p.44)

Vitamin C

Vitamin C is essential for tissue repair, wound healing, bone growth and repair, and healthy skin. Vitamin C also helps your body to fight infection and it acts as an antioxidant, protecting cells from damage.

Foods high in vitamin C are: citrus fruits and green vegetables. Try drinking orange juice at the same meal as eating iron-rich food to maximise your iron intake.

Zinc

Zinc is essential for the production, repair and functioning of DNA, the body's genetic blueprint and the basis for cell formation.

Good sources of zinc are: meat, seafood, eggs, fermented soya products such as tempeh and miso, wholegrains, nuts, seeds and some fortified cereals.

Omega-3 fatty acids

Omega-3 fatty acids are essential and can only be obtained from diet. These are critical for the brain development of your babies.

Good sources of omega-3 fatty acids are: fish with low mercury levels, such as salmon, sardines and mackerel, corn oil, soya oil, egg yolks, meat and spinach. The current dietary advice is to have two servings of fish a week, one of which should be an oily fish, such as salmon, trout, herrings or sardines.

Fibre

Fibre is good for digestion and for avoiding constipation. If you are starting to add more fibre to your diet, do so slowly and remember to increase your fluid intake, too, otherwise, ironically, you will become constipated.

Good sources of fibre are: fruit, vegetables, wholegrains and dried fruits, especially dried apricots and prunes.

Peanuts

Advice about eating peanuts during pregnancy has changed. Unless you have a peanut allergy or a health professional has advised you not to eat them, there is no evidence that eating peanuts during pregnancy increases the chances of your babies having a peanut allergy. If you are concerned about allergies relating to other nuts or any other food, talk to your GP for more specific advice.

Things to avoid during pregnancy

You should cut out the following from your diet while you are pregnant: mould-ripened cheeses such as blue cheese and Camembert, raw fish, shellfish and raw or partially cooked eggs.

It is not necessary to go without caffeine entirely, but NHS guidelines suggest limiting yourself to about 200 mg a day. A mug of filter coffee is about 140 mg of caffeine, a mug of tea is 75 mg and a can of cola is 40 mg.

Advice on what level of alcohol is safe during pregnancy can be a little confusing. However, official guidelines suggest that until there is a definitive position, you should err on the side of caution and refrain from drinking any alcohol at all. Research shows that drinking alcohol, particularly in the first three months of your pregnancy, increases the risk of a premature birth and low birth weight. Heavy drinking can result in foetal alcohol syndrome, which results in your babies having learning difficulties, facial abnormalities and poor growth.

By not smoking during pregnancy, you will reduce the chances of your babies being born underweight, reduce the risk of sudden infant death syndrome (previously known as cot death) and increase the likelihood of having a healthier, more straightforward pregnancy. Cigarettes can reduce your babies' oxygen supply, so their hearts have to beat faster every time you smoke. For all of those reasons, smoking during pregnancy is not recommended.

Snacks

Suggestions for portable and nutritional snacks:

▶ Fruit – one of the easiest, healthiest and most portable snacks which will provide you with vitamins, minerals and help your digestion too. Try frozen (good for making smoothies), canned, juiced or dried fruit as well as fresh for extra variety.

▶ Flapjack – It is easy to make, lasts for a long time and you can throw in nuts, chopped dried fruit and seeds for even more goodness.

▶ Sandwiches – Don't think of these only as lunchtime fodder – they are perfect to have on hand at any time when hunger strikes. Good-quality, high-protein fillings – such as slices of hard-boiled egg, lean meat and cheese with chopped walnuts – are great pick-me-ups.

▶ Breakfast cereal – But not necessarily just at breakfast; cereals are usually fortified with vitamins and minerals. Choose low sugar varieties and avoid those coated in sugar.

▶ Hummus with vegetable sticks, bread sticks, oatcakes or pitta bread. This chickpea snack is rich in protein and is a good way of combating hunger cravings. Veggie sticks on their own are great too – colourful and crunch slices of cucumber, pepper and carrot are ideal.

▶ Nuts and seeds – These are good sources of essential fatty acids as well as fibre, protein and minerals. Almonds, cashews, peanuts, walnuts or pistachios are high in fat but provide a hefty dose of vitamins and minerals. The same applies to seeds such as pumpkin, sesame or sunflower seeds. Whilst nuts are healthy for many reasons they are energy dense so eat in moderation to avoid gaining too much weight.

▶ Popcorn – In its simplest form this is low in calories and contains antioxidants which help fight disease. But beware – many shop-bought versions are coated in sugar or toffee which should be avoided. Popping your own is the healthiest option.

▶ Yoghurt – This is a great source of calcium and protein and can be combined with pureed fruit or berries or just eaten plain for a great snack.

&&I took my diet seriously as I felt it was a way of helping the babies reach a good birth weight. It is such a feat for our bodies to produce two babies – you have to eat a bit like an athlete! &&

Susanne, mum to Delphie and Isadora, 22 months; Nicolas, five; and Ana-Marie, six

&&I did try to be super healthy because I was paranoid about the babies being small – if you have extra doughnuts it doesn't help them in any way, so I tried to have very healthy food. &&

Katie, mum to Keira and Gracie, 11 months; and Layla, five

Exercise

Keeping exercise regimes going is generally recommended during pregnancy. A reasonable level of fitness helps you adapt better to your changing body and weight, cope more easily with labour and should also benefit you as you try to return to your pre-pregnancy size after birth. Moderate activities such as swimming, walking and cycling on an exercise bike (which is less likely to result in a fall than normal cycling) are recommended. If you have a more vigorous exercise programme, it may be possible to continue this during your pregnancy, but discuss it with your doctor first.

It's never too early for pelvic floor exercises – particularly if you have any plans to sneeze or laugh again post-birth. You can feel your pelvic muscles when you stop your urine mid flow. One simple exercise (when you aren't mid flow) is to squeeze your pelvic floor muscles 10–15 times in a row without holding your breath or tightening your stomach muscles.

66 I had to switch from running to Pilates very early on and then had to give that up when I couldn't get up off the couch. I had everything that I'd experienced with my first pregnancy – just magnified tenfold. 99

Adwoa, mum to Ti-Jean, six; Maui and Loki, two

Being the centre of attention

In addition to your worries about complications, previously unheard of conditions and a whole load of new vitamins to get to grips with, your body image issues may well have taken on a life of their own.

Your feet are a distant memory, you can't sleep and you need an extra shove just to make it out of bed in the morning. In an ideal world, you would heave yourself quietly through the minimum of activity and hope that no one has noticed your elephantine presence at the local shop. Unluckily for you, that ain't going to happen.

Perhaps the constant – and, frankly, sometimes intrusive – interest your bump attracts is just nature's way of preparing you for the barrage of attention you will face once your twins arrive.

Strangers' hands will find their way to your bump, people will point and stare and, yes, the occasional mobile phone will record your great size. Somewhere on social media, people you have never met in countries you have never visited may be discussing your enormity.

66 Everybody thinks that they are the biggest thing ever when they were pregnant, but I really was. I was enormous. People I knew just didn't know what to say. A stranger stopped me and said: 'How are you going to push that out?'. I went from just under 8 stone to 11 stone. Bending down to pick something up required me to psyche myself up. I had to be efficient — if I was going to bend down I had to make sure I picked up everything I was likely to need for a few hours in one go. I got very breathless and often felt dizzy just from going up and down stairs. 99

Lucy, mum to Jack and Iona, five months; Beth, five; and Sam, three

66 People stopped me in the street all the time which was very tedious. I suppose the only good thing was that I was pregnant with twins. A woman passed me in the street and literally stopped in her tracks and said: 'Oh my god, this woman's expecting twins. Can you believe she's even standing?'

On the days leading up to when the babies were delivered I felt sluggish, almost a bit stoned — I couldn't focus and needed a nap all the time. On the last day I couldn't even raise my arms. 99

Alicia, mum to Penny and Abe, six months

Learning to cope with this attention is difficult but essential. Responding for the hundredth time to a cheery 'Not long to go now!' when you're only five months pregnant requires considerable acting aplomb. Usually an attempt at a smile and an untruthful 'yes!' will suffice, but some people will insist on following up inane openers with even more banal observations – none of them likely to be flattering – so picking up the pace slightly, reaching for your phone or spotting an imaginary friend in the distance to wave at can all be useful tactics for breaking eye contact and, hopefully, further interrogation.

Most people's interest is perfectly natural, friendly and well meaning, and some women enjoy sharing their joy at carrying twins. However, the peak of the public's interest tends to come at a time when you are tired and probably anxious about the babies' impending birth, as well as feeling very self-conscious about your size. Being made to feel like a freak show act does not help. If the attention is really getting you down, channel your inner celebrity and keep your public at bay by putting on headphones, dark glasses and a pout when you venture out.

Work, maternity leave and paternity leave

Most women want to work as close to their due date as possible in order to maximise their time at home with their babies, but planning your leave when your health and that of your twins is so uncertain makes this a very difficult calculation. Allow for the fact that you are working back from 37 weeks, rather than 40, and that even if your pregnancy is straightforward, you will be bigger and more tired than if you were carrying one baby.

You are required to notify your employer of your pregnancy, your due date and the date you wish to start your maternity leave at least 15 weeks before your babies are due. Your midwife will give you a form that confirms your due date and which you pass on to your employer.

Once your employer knows you are pregnant, you are entitled to attend antenatal appointments during working hours. Your partner is also entitled to accompany you to two antenatal appointments. It will be assumed that you will take your full 52 weeks' maternity leave. If you want to return before that time, you need to give your employer eight weeks' notice.

You are entitled to sick leave during your pregnancy, although it is recommended that pregnancy-related sick days should be recorded separately to ordinary sick leave so that the absence is not used as a reason for disciplinary action, dismissal or redundancy. If your sick leave coincides with the period in which your statutory maternity pay is calculated then it may affect the amount of maternity pay you receive.

If you are off sick with a pregnancy-related illness in the last four weeks of pregnancy, your employer can start your maternity leave, even if you are off sick for only one day. However, if you are ill for just a short time, your employer may agree to let you start your maternity leave when you had planned.

If your baby is born early, your maternity leave and statutory maternity pay will start on the day after the birth.

Paternity leave of up to two weeks is available to fathers (biological and adoptive), husbands, civil partners, and partners of either sex who live with the mother in a family relationship. This cannot start before the birth and must end within 56 days of the birth. You do not need to give your employers a precise date when you want to take leave, but can specify a general time, such as the day of the birth or a week after the birth. You need to give your employer 28 days' notice if you want to change your start date.

Chapter 5

Help and Where to Find It

One of the most overused pieces of advice given to new parents of twins is to accept whatever help is going. Although offers of help may be sprayed around liberally in the run-up to your twins' arrival, selecting the right level of assistance from the right people needs careful thought and ambassadorial levels of tact.

The perfect helpers – whether it be family, friends or someone you pay – will make your life easier, lift some of the more mundane chores from your shoulders and allow you to get on with looking after your family. The wrong kind of helper, however, will add to your anxiety with unwanted advice and judgements, diverting valuable energy from your main task of caring for your twins.

Family members hope to fall into the first category, but often thud into the second. Equally, if professional caregivers are not chosen well, they can be imposing and intimidating. Ideally, your helpers will bolster your morale, act on their own initiative in terms of understanding what needs to be done, respect your choices, keep you fed and watered and remind you how well you are doing.

With budgets already stretched to the max, drafting in paid help of any kind may feel like a huge extravagance, which is why so many of us rely on our family and friends to help us get through those difficult early weeks. However, not everyone is lucky enough to have family who are local, or indeed available, to come and look after you for weeks on end. Whatever your financial situation, planning the help you think you will need well in advance will help to focus your mind on what needs to be done and who is best placed to support you.

Everyone's reaction to help is different – some people are so grateful to have an extra pair of hands that they are happy to overlook irritating habits, while others find the presence of extra people in their house stressful and are unable to let go of looking after guests' welfare.

66 I hate being 'helped' with things, and there was a kind of assumption that I would never cope on my own, which meant that there were people around me all the time which was awful... and conversely made me completely unable to ask for help when I needed it as I had spent so long declaring that we were doing just fine on our own. I think twins, more so than other babies, are kind of considered public property and I really wanted to be left on my own with them, in the big bed, with some snacks, just to look at them and smell them and kiss them. I didn't want people coming and 'giving me a break' by taking them away, but that's really all people want to do. My husband works shifts and nights, so we were on our own a lot or relying on grandparents... which is nice but awful at the same time. 99

Lindsay, mum to Alex and Serafina, 22 months

66 A woman who I knew from walking the dog offered to give me a hand when the twins were born. She couldn't ever remember my name but asked for my number, which she said she'd remember – I never thought she would. On the twins' due date she left a voicemail asking if they had arrived, I couldn't believe it. She used to come round once a week and help me at lunchtime – it was lovely. I felt so grateful that my twins gave so many other people so much joy. 99

Meryl, mum to Harri and Gethin, seven

When you are considering what help you will need, draw up a list of close friends or family who are likely to be available and who you would feel comfortable with in your house. If people who have offered to help do not make it on to the guest list, give them something to do that does not involve them spending too much time at your house, such as preparing a weekly meal, taking a load of ironing home or taking an older child out for the afternoon.

After you have worked out the extent of your 'free' help, decide whether you can afford to buy in any additional assistance. Paid help options start from a cleaner and go up to a maternity nurse or nanny (see later in the chapter). Whatever the price tag, help is only useful if you find the right person, which requires research and an interview process so give yourself enough time to get this in place well before the babies are due.

Self-help

There are a few things you can do in advance to make life easier once your twins arrive, which mainly involve clearing the decks of any outstanding jobs, trying to anticipate the demands of the early days with the babies and filling your freezer with food. Warning: if you are not a particularly organised person, look away now.

Self-help tips:

▶ Depending on your levels of culinary expertise, make large batches of your favourite meals (such as Bolognese sauce, fish pies or casseroles) and freeze them into individual or double portions. When the babies are home you probably will not feel like cooking, so being able to defrost a good meal will make life a lot easier. If you don't want to cook, stock up on plenty of your favourite freezable meals.

▶ If you have older children, be really generous with play dates now (if you've got the energy for them), so that when your twins arrive you've got plenty owing and you'll feel less guilty about farming your little ones out to friends.

▶ Organise your finances. With extra equipment to buy and a possible drop in income once the babies arrive, work out how much you will have to spend each month. Are any major bills due? Could you switch to direct debits to avoid the chances of forgetting to pay them? Submit your tax return.

▶ Go for a sight test and get your hair cut. Visit the dentist for free – you are entitled to free NHS dental treatment if you are pregnant when you're accepted for a course of treatment. Get up to date with anything else you know is likely to come up within a few months of the twins' birth.

▶ If you do Internet food shopping, set up a 'saved' shopping list to make it even quicker.

▶ If you are someone who will be upset if you forget birthdays, go through your calendar for the next three months and buy cards and stamps for each birthday. The only flaw in this plan is that you still have to remember to send them. If you have older children who may be attending birthday parties, stock up on a few generic kids' birthday cards and emergency presents to avoid a last-minute panic.

Family

If you have the option, drafting in family members is the obvious first port of call when considering help. Not only do your close relatives know you best, and are therefore likely to be more tolerant of the occasional parental meltdown, but they are also free and come with a huge vested interest in your lovely new twins.

However, give potential family helpers a lot of thought before your twins arrive and be clear of the role each family member will take on.

A few tips for making family help a success:

► Play to each person's strengths. If your mother-in-law is a fantastic cook but a little over zealous with her advice giving, ask her to take charge of the family's meals during her stay. If your brother is not really a baby person, get him to drive you to appointments or have a list of jobs ready (assembling new equipment, keeping the garden under control, taking an older child out).

► Be realistic about what they can do and give them some respite. Helping is hard work, especially if your parents are elderly.

► Have a rota of helpers (siblings and parents, if possible) taking it in turns to stop anyone becoming too annoying or tired. Have a weekend team for people who want to help but who work or aren't available during the week.

► Be clear about what you want them to do. Don't feel embarrassed about asking someone to cook or clean – most people are glad to feel useful.

► Be honest with yourself about the areas that are likely to cause friction and try to work out a way of coping with it beforehand. Family can get under your skin like no one else. Does it really matter if your mother-in-law irons your husband's underpants? If it does, hide the iron.

66 We were lucky enough to be surrounded by a wonderful family who came and helped when they could. Everyone had their limitations in what they could do but with a bit of coordination grandparents and aunts and uncles all experienced the special joys that twins bring to a family. It just so happened that my mum was happy to do night feeds whereas my mother-in-law preferred to look after us during the day. It was a good combination! On the luxurious days that I had both Grandmas around I got a full night's sleep. Even one or two days of rest like that made all the difference to the rest of the week. 99

Sabreena, mum to Nadia and Yasmin, seven

66 Eventually you get fed up of eating cold curry and rubbish. My mum used to bring us round a few meals a week, which was great and if we were cooking we'd make extra so we could freeze the leftovers. When my parents or my wife's best friend were due to come over they would always text us beforehand and see if we needed anything picking up on the way, which really helped. 99

Daniel, dad to Sophie and Hannah, three

Friends

Friends tend to come with a lot less baggage than family and can be lifesavers simply by bringing you up to date with life in the outside world or by allowing you to have a good, uninterrupted moan.

It is often easier to ask friends to do jobs, such as cook a meal or bring over some shopping, although if they haven't got children (or even if they have) you may feel they don't fully understand how tired you are and how relentlessly demanding life with twins can be.

66 I did feel a bit trapped at home when the boys were tiny babies. It was a hot summer and the flat was like a sweat box. Even going into the garden seemed a palaver as we had steps to it. Friends would visit but we tended to stay in. With hindsight I wish I'd asked them for a bit of help in getting out and about – just to go somewhere for a cup of tea and some cake would have helped. 99

Milly, mum to Alfred and Joseph, two

Home-Start

Home-Start is a charity that supports families in practical ways in their home setting. It can be invaluable for parents of twins, as a volunteer can be arranged to help out for a few hours a week. Volunteers are all parents themselves and are trained and checked before being carefully allocated to their family. They may help you to attend an appointment, be a shoulder to cry on, assist you in getting to a local playgroup or give advice if you ask for it. Although they will not assume sole care of the children, the volunteer will help you as well as offer encouragement.

66 When my twins were six months old we moved house. My then husband was working away from home Monday to Friday so I was on my own with three children aged two and under, with no friends and no family to help. My Home-Start volunteer would come every Wednesday for two to three hours and was my lifeline. If I hadn't had her, I don't think I would ever have had the confidence to leave the house. She

would look after the children while I had a shower or caught up on some sleep, or other times she would listen and we'd discuss any problems that had come up. She encouraged me to go to a family group that Home-Start ran and went with me until I had the confidence to take the three of them on my own. I met people there who were in exactly my situation and they are still my friends now. 〞

Claire, mum to Corey and Miriam, five; Kara, seven; and Malcolm, seven months

See the Resources and Further Reading chapter for details of how to find out if Home-Start operates in your area.

Cleaner

There can be no better excuse to abandon cleaning entirely than becoming the parents of twins. The only problem being that dust, debris and general rubbish tend to accumulate even more rapidly with two extra people in the house, making it hard to ignore the issue entirely. Being surrounded by low-level filth is not all it's cracked up to be, so some parents of twins invest in a cleaner, even if only for a few weeks. It may seem like a luxury at a time when your finances are stretched already, but it can make life a lot more comfortable – so long as you can clear sufficient space for the cleaner to make a difference.

Mother's help

A rather old-fashioned term, but mother's help can be a relatively affordable way of getting a break. If you are lucky enough to have a sensible teenager as a neighbour or have a college nearby that offers childcare, you may be able to draft in somebody enthusiastic, reliable and cheap for a few hours a day to help during stressful periods. Friends with young children may be able to recommend their babysitter or someone trustworthy to help on an ad hoc basis. Many mothers find it a godsend to have an extra pair of hands at bath time, over lunchtime or at naptime to allow them to switch off and sleep, too. This type of help may involve more supervision and you may not be comfortable, at least initially, in leaving your helper in sole care of the babies, but just having someone to share tasks with can provide a much-needed break.

> 66 I limped on until they were about four months and then I thought 'I can't do this any more'. I had a student who came round for three hours over lunchtime so that I could get some sleep. I was really resistant to the idea because I felt like I wasn't earning money so this was my job and I should be able to do it on my own, but the reality is that it can send you over the edge. When I think about it now though, I realise that, ironically, I arranged the hours of childcare around Hannah, the student, and not me! 99
>
> *Pip, mum to Bertie and Polly, two; and Charlie, 12 months*

Postnatal doula

The word 'doula' (pronounced doola) literally means 'slave' or 'woman who serves'. A doula's job is to put you, the mother, at the centre of her work. She will do whatever you need to help you focus on your babies and ensure that you get as much rest as possible. She will cook, take other siblings to school or entertain young ones while you are resting as well as tidying up, putting on the laundry, ironing clothes and taking on whatever tasks need doing to make your life easier. She will also be able to help and advise you on feeding, but should be respectful of whatever choices you make in terms of breast or bottle-feeding.

Although doula regulation is not a legal requirement, there is a central organisation for doulas called Doula UK and this is the best place to find people local to you. The mother–doula relationship is a very personal one and it is your responsibility to make a judgement on a doula's experience and suitability for your home life. Women who become doulas often have midwifery experience or come to the profession having had children themselves. There is no formal qualification, but a woman must be mentored by a proficient doula and gain a certain level of experience herself before she is recognised by Doula UK. Doulas can also help with antenatal care and/or support during birth. Although the vast majority of doulas are women, there are a few male doulas (sometimes known as 'dude-las') who carry out the same role.

❝ I knew from having my first daughter that I would not get the support I needed from my family. For us, we had to balance need against financial affordability. My husband took on an extra freelance job so that we could afford a doula. She came twice a week for a minimum of four hours – once in the morning and once in the evening. She would always make us good food to eat in the evening on the days that she came. She had her own key and would just get on if I was asleep. She was so aware of what needed to be done, there was no need to manage her or think about it. She dealt with the laundry, cleaning and food but was also this emotional blanket who allowed me to feel that I was doing alright – she made me feel like I was doing a great job. ❞

Yasmeen, mum to Khalil and Eesa, three; and Hanifah, 11

Nanny

A nanny either lives in or, more commonly, lives out. In most circumstances they will be employed permanently either full time or part time. Unless you share a nanny, you will employ them and therefore are responsible for checking they are allowed to work in the UK, providing them with a contract, giving them payslips and ensuring they are paid at least the national minimum wage. Nannies are entitled to maternity pay, sick pay, paid holiday and redundancy pay. If you share a nanny, however, they may be self-employed, in which case you are not required to register as their employer.

Red tape aside, a nanny will provide a full range of childcare, including cooking for children, taking them out and about, and tidying up after them. They may perform light housework duties and run errands, but this would have to be clarified beforehand. A nanny's role is to look after children, not adults, so their care will not extend to you.

Selecting a nanny is a very personal decision. Your nanny is likely to have a very close relationship with your children, which can spark understandable jealousy if you have to work long hours or away from home. Although it is crucial that they establish a great rapport with your twins, you need to be able to work well together and trust each other completely.

> ❝ We knew that we needed a nanny as we were both going to be working full-time. There was nothing particularly wrong with the candidates that the agencies sent – I just didn't get the right feeling from any of them. I suppose it was a bit like going on lots of blind dates – for months, I despaired of the candidates I met (ranging from the slightly annoying to

completely bizarre), then I decided to advertise on Gumtree. Cue literally hundreds of weirdos and somewhere amongst them... Esme.

Esme didn't have any twin experience, was only 23 and lived in Germany, but her reply to the ad had something very caring and mature about it. We had a Skype interview and got on very well – during the interview she asked me various questions about how I treat the twins, which no one else had asked.

Four years on and she is still with us – she has fitted in perfectly and the twins have no idea that she's not a family member. I think we have been amazingly lucky.

My advice would be to treat the process as a job interview – take your time to pick the right person and be guided by your instincts. Anyone can look good on paper, but you really need to meet them and see how they get on with the kids. 🌝

Jan, mum to Jamie and Sophia, five

Independent midwife

It is a brave woman who opts for a home birth with twins (see Chapter 7 for one such example). This decision will not be supported by the NHS, so to even begin this process you will need to engage the services of an independent midwife. An independent midwife is a fully qualified midwife who has chosen to work outside the NHS. She will carry out antenatal appointments, check your blood pressure and urine samples, and monitor the development of the baby, as well as supervise your birth and the first few weeks with your twin babies. She is able to offer continuity of care that many women do not experience through the NHS, and can be flexible about appointments, often coming to your home in the evenings or at weekends.

Independent midwives are regulated by the Nursing & Midwifery Council and are subject to the same supervision as NHS midwives. An independent midwife is self-employed and must hold professional indemnity insurance.

Maternity nurse

Unless you have very deep pockets, this tends to be a short-term option, often triggered by extreme sleep deprivation and desperation. Maternity nurses are trained or experienced nurses or nannies who specialise in the care of newborn babies. Their help begins when you leave hospital, and lasts until you and the babies are settled into a routine at home.

You can employ a maternity nurse to be 'on call' over a 24-hour period or you can use her services on a 'day-only' or 'night-only' basis. The number of hours or days you require is flexible depending on how much you can afford or need (alas, the two don't usually tally). A maternity nurse is self-employed.

Au pair

This can often seem like a cost-effective option, but needs to be thought through carefully. An au pair is a young foreign adult who would live in your home and help with light housework and childcare in return for a rent-free room, free meals and a chance to learn English with your family, as well as time to attend English language classes. They would expect to receive 'pocket money' of £70–£85 a week. An au pair would live in your house, but is not classed as an employee and is not entitled to the national minimum wage or paid holidays. An au pair is not officially employed by you (unlike a nanny) and therefore you are not liable for providing standard benefits.

There are many au pair agencies that can put you in touch with candidates and you can choose to interview via Skype to ensure you get the right person.

Unless you are really lucky, it is probably unrealistic to expect your au pair to take the initiative with either childcare or cleaning so you will have to oversee their help and it may take a while to build your relationship, particularly as there may be a language barrier to contend with, too. Parents often turn to au pairs towards the end of their first year, when a routine is more established and it is easier to manage a rather needy stranger in the house.

Finally, no matter how useful their help is, there will come a time when you want everyone out of your house so that you can concentrate on raising your own family in your own way.

Chapter 6

Twins and Your Family

Firstborns are brought up with the unquestioning belief that Mummy and Daddy exist only to cater for their every whim, lavish them with love and attention, and tell them how clever they are. So when two new siblings are simultaneously parachuted into the family and the realisation dawns that these noisy brothers and sisters are also entitled to all of the above, it is not surprising that excitement can quickly turn to resentment.

Children aren't the only ones affected by the new arrivals. Even the strongest adult relationship can face a buffeting as couples compete with each other over who has had the least sleep or worked the hardest. Remembering that you're on the same side (or even that you quite like each other) can sometimes be difficult. It is no wonder that research shows parents of twins are more likely to find their relationship under strain and have a greater chance of divorce than parents of single children.

Before their arrival, invest in some time to imagine life with your twins, to discuss how you can twin-proof your adult relationship and to talk to your existing children, no matter how young, about the changes their new siblings are likely to bring about. This preparation can go some way towards lessening the impact of their appearance.

Let the countdown begin!
Preparing an older child for the arrival of twin siblings may feel a bit like telling them that one day the world will be made of ice cream. It's a momentous and exciting piece of news, but it hasn't

happened yet, so... 'Hmmm, where can I stick this piece of Play-Doh?'

Even if your older child seems too small to understand the upcoming event or doesn't appear particularly interested in the news, it is never too early to lay the groundwork for the family changes that are afoot.

Children's books about the arrival of new twins are fairly thin on the ground but you can use stories about an impending new baby, or babies, to prompt a conversation with your child about what life will be like with twins at home. (See the Resources and Further Reading chapter for book recommendations.) Talk with your child or children about the fact that you will be in hospital, and that the babies will often cry and will sometimes take up a lot of everyone's attention. At the same time, keep the talk about the new babies positive and reassure them that they will continue to be loved as much as ever and will always be special in the eyes of Mum, Dad and the new babies.

❝ You should start talking to your older child about the arrival of twins as soon as possible and to help them understand that life is really going to change, but that your love is not finite. It is not like a chocolate cake where the more people want it, the less you get, it is like having lots and lots of different chocolate cakes. Enough for everyone. Life will be difficult but there will be good things as well as bad things. Parents need to let their existing children know that it is going to be tough and that Mummy is going to be stressed and teary sometimes. ❞

Dr Sarah Helps, consultant clinical psychologist and family therapist, and mum to 12-year-old twins

> ❝ Ben was only 18 months when the girls were born so was too young to understand much, which now I feel was good because he doesn't really remember anything else. We encouraged him to talk to Mummy's tummy and he used to blow raspberries on it. One of the best things I did was to buy him a doll from a charity shop, which he really enjoyed playing with. When the girls came home he could carry on looking after his doll – including trying to breastfeed her! ❞
>
> *Emma, mum to Amelie and Jessica, 23 months;*
> *and Ben, three*

When the babies arrive

The period surrounding your twins' birth can be especially difficult for your other children. If you have had an unexpected complication, you may have disappeared into hospital with no warning, which can be frightening for young children who take for granted that you will be around at certain key points of the day, such as bedtime. If the pregnancy has gone to term, you may be very tired and sluggish and, although you are still at home, you may feel guilty that you simply do not have the energy to play with your children in the way you used to.

If the twins have been born early and are in special care, there are decisions to be made about how to introduce your children in a way that is not upsetting and does not make them anxious. Visiting the babies in hospital can present parents with a dilemma in terms of how much to prepare their children for the experience. Children can be better at looking past the beeps and the wires in hospital than adults, who understandably bring their baggage and worries to the scene. Some child psychologists suggest a minimum of preparation beforehand, and for parents to answer the questions their children ask as a consequence of their particular visit rather than pre-empting how they may feel.

A few tips for easy ways to assist your older children in adjusting to the new babies:

▶ Arrange for the new babies to 'give' their older sibling a present to celebrate their arrival.

▶ Make a fuss about the older children being the 'first' to do certain activities, such as holding the babies, choosing their coming-home outfits or selecting their first cuddly toy.

▶ Involve the older children so that they feel proud of helping without making them responsible for the babies. For example, they could stand by mum passing nappies or could put their hands in the bath to make little waves to entertain the babies. When mum goes for a wee they could be 'in charge' of singing to the babies to entertain them.

▶ Make time for your older child. With two babies to look after, this is very hard. Sometimes this will mean ignoring your crying twins for a few minutes while you finish building a tower or playing a game. This sends a clear message that you still value your time together.

▶ Put yourself in their position. Ask yourself: how would I feel if this were me? Acknowledge the disruption the twins have caused to family life from your child's perspective.

Please note: be careful about giving older children too much responsibility – encourage any help that is volunteered, but any involvement in the babies' care should be through choice.

❝ The twins don't know any different: they have always been twins, and they have always had an older sibling. In contrast, the older child may have been an only child and will miss the time he or she had alone with you.

Try not to 'fix' peoples' emotions. If your older child has just had their Lego tower knocked over by the younger children and has reacted by bashing them over the head, try not to take sides. It is tempting to tell the older child that they shouldn't get cross because the twins are only little. However, having your Lego tower knocked over when you're still only small – or big! – is horrid. It is OK to say, 'I can see that's made you really cross. Come on, I'll help you to rebuild it.' ❞

Dr Bonamy Oliver, developmental psychologist with special expertise in twin families

❝ I felt I was always telling Joseph to 'just wait a minute, wait a minute', because I was always feeding one baby and even if someone came to help me, I still had one baby in my arms – I was never able to be on my own with him. It was almost harder when they got more mobile as they'd crawl through his jigsaws or knock over his tower and, to him, that was the end of the world. It was hard for Joseph – it must have been so annoying to have these little wrecking balls come along, break your jigsaw and then chew the pieces. I had a travel cot with toys in it, which I used as a play pen, so I'd put Ben and Finlay in there if I needed to keep them separate. Also, we lived in a bungalow so I could help Joseph lay out something to play with and then close the baby gate so it couldn't be disturbed by the babies. However, the fact that he's older means he has the trump card because he is allowed to do things that they aren't, so I think that makes having twin brothers a bit easier. ❞

Gillian, mum to Benjamin and Finlay, three; and Joseph, five

    When the babies arrived we put a 'present' from them in their cots in the hospital – Rosie gave our older son a little teddy bear and Elliott gave him a packet of chocolate buttons. Whether it was due to bribery or not, he took to them straight away. He was of the age where he liked to help, so when we changed their nappies, he'd be the one who passed up each wipe or sometimes we'd have a guessing game of 'is there going to be a poo or not going to be a poo'. Just little things, but we talked to him a lot about what was happening and tried to make it fun. We may just have been lucky, but so far it seems to have worked.

James, dad to Rosie and Elliott, seven months; and Robin, three

Don't underestimate the effect the change in family circumstances will have on you, too. Being deprived of special, fun time with your older child can be hard and you may feel very guilty at watching your son or daughter being packed off to the childminder or taken to the park by friends instead of you. Try to give yourself and your older child some time together, too, even if it's just a few minutes when the babies are occupied or asleep.

    I made a packed lunch for my daughter and kept it on the lowest shelf in the fridge so she could help herself when I was feeding the boys. I cried my eyes out as I watched her getting it out, remembering when we'd sit and have lunch together, just the two of us.

Sarah, mum to Alex and Jake, six; and Nell, nine

Naturally, introducing two, noisy strangers into the household is rarely a seamless process, and suddenly being a sibling to twins isn't always easy. Tantrums and heavy-handedness around the babies is common. Try not to let the age of the babies artificially inflate the maturity of your older child in your mind. It is easy to forget that your older child or children may still be very young and may not understand how fragile babies are. Even if all they want to do is kiss and cuddle new siblings, it's sensible to supervise your older child with the babies to make sure they don't hurt them.

66 It is not uncommon for existing children to try to hurt the new babies. Give them a clear message not to hit and don't leave them together, but try a 'show and tell' approach. Talk about being kind and gentle, do something with all three of them so you can show them how to be with small babies. Ask them to use 'kind' hands and not 'hurty' hands. Acknowledge the pain – your three year old might be sensitive to noise and find the babies' crying really difficult. Have a conversation about how annoying it is. 99

Dr Sarah Helps, consultant clinical psychologist and family therapist, and mum to 12-year-old twins

66 Sibling conflict can be hard to watch as a parent, but it is good for children! It is a way to learn how to deal with conflict in a space of safety. That's why siblings can be so grotty towards each other in a way they would probably not be with anyone else.

When it comes to sibling relationships, try to allow them to be what they will be if you can. In particular, be prepared for relationships between the children to change. At various points it might seem like one child will have a better relationship with one sibling than another, or that the twins will be particularly 'twinny', but the wheel will spin and it will change again and again. Try not to intervene to even up relationships or make sure everyone is included. If you let them be, you'll most likely find that different members of the sibling group are close at different times. It is so much more about creating a loving environment where people feel they have individual relationships with family members and are appreciated for who they are. 🔊

Dr Bonamy Oliver, developmental psychologist with special expertise in twin families

Twin-proofing your adult relationship

One of the hopeful claims made about having children is that it helps to cement your adult relationship. Certainly, the joy of producing these two lovely babies is a uniting force, but the additional pressure of having very little sleep, time, sex, conversation and often money can temporarily reduce your partnership to a husk of its former self.

Finding time for each other as well as the babies, existing children and work can seem like a step too far in a day that is already stretched to breaking point.

🔊 The couple relationship can be put under enormous stress. There is probably not going to be very much sex and there is probably not going to be much sleep. Couples are likely to be irritable with each other, especially if one partner is at work all day then comes home and feels like they need to put their feet up when you've been stuck in with two babies. Being kind to each other as a couple is absolutely vital. Try to have time together without the babies if it's possible, perhaps go out together every few weeks, once the babies are about six months. It doesn't have to be for an expensive meal – it might be a walk around the park or a quick pint. 🙶

Dr Sarah Helps, consultant clinical psychologist and family therapist, and mum to 12-year-old twins

Tips for easing the strain on your adult relationship:

► Before the babies arrive, talk about your expectations of parenthood and about what you want to do when the twins get here.

► Talk about your own childhoods and the messages you remember from your own families about how infants and babies should be treated.

► If you can't go out together, stay in and have a takeaway. Agree not to talk about the children.

► Give each other a break – it's not a competition. If your partner has gone back to work then the chances are he or she will be getting up in the night, doing a full day at the office and then returning home to have a crying baby plonked into their arms and, possibly, a sobbing partner on their shoulder. You are both working really hard. Draft in family members or friends to give each other a few hours off.

66 What's really important is that you have to have a strong relationship because having twins tests you. It either makes you stronger or ruins you for life! I'd say, try to keep talking and respect each other, and if you do snap at each other (and you will), don't take it personally – if you've only had two hours' sleep that's just how it is. 99

Daniel, dad to Hannah and Sophie, three; and Michael 12

66 We had a crunch at five weeks. We both got the norovirus and my mum had to come and help, which was not much help as it turned out. We just couldn't cope and at one point my boyfriend walked out. I had a vision of me being a single mum to twins. It was awful.

When the babies were 11 weeks we hired a cottage in North Wales with my partner's mum and sister. We didn't really do very much, but it was great just getting away and not having to do all the other rubbish that you have to deal with at home. A change of scene was great and really helped us all. 99

Alison, mum to Sylvie and Mila, 12 months

66 My son took to breastfeeding, my daughter not so much. So we fell into a pattern that my partner would feed Mattie and I would feed Evie. We felt like two single parents who lived together. 99

Darren, dad to Mattie and Evie, ten: Eliza three

What about me... ?

Yes, you! That person who may have been financially independent, had lots of energy, possibly quite a lot of sex and had the ability to do things on impulse (even if you rarely actually did them).

Life with baby twins can seem like a treadmill of feeding, washing, nappy changing, crying and more feeding. Even with the wonderful bursts of sunshine that your babies are likely to bring you every day, there is no escaping the fact that this is hard graft, with very little respite.

> 66 The problem at the moment is having time for the rest of life. I had one of those days this week – my husband put a nappy on badly so poo suddenly spurted everywhere, then I opened a cupboard and a jar of olives in brine smashed on the floor. I had to phone a neighbour and ask her to take my daughter to school. I suddenly thought 'Oh My God, there is never any time. I've got the twins, my older daughter, my writing, the washing, the cleaning – it just never stops.' That is the challenge at the moment. 99
>
> *Katie, mum to Keira and Gracie, 11 months; and Layla, five*

> 66 I am mum to the older two, mum to the twins, I have the house to look after, I'm a daughter – with my parents quite reliant on me – and a wife and then there's Laura, who's a tiny, tiny speck. I do sometimes think I would love five minutes with the old Laura – that's the biggest challenge, losing me in the midst of the big family. 99
>
> *Laura, mum to Heidi and Rory, ten months; Lewis, three; and Niamh, five*

And finally...

Nobody is perfect. You are likely to shout, rage, pound your chest (and possibly others' chests, too), cry, say things you don't mean, doubt your ability to be a competent mother or father and generally skid off the parental rails a few times. This is normal. Bad days may seem like they're coming thick and fast in the beginning, but, as you all get used to your new reality, life will become easier. Don't be too hard on yourself and give yourself time and space. Try to be as compassionate with yourself as you would be with a friend in the same boat.

> Parenting can feel like the most important job in the world... but it is not the end of the world if you get things wrong sometimes. If you are sensitive to your children's needs, you love them and care for them, you're doing a great job. Don't beat yourself up over every mistake. We all make them.
>
> *Dr Bonamy Oliver, developmental psychologist with special expertise in twin families*

Chapter 7

Birth

No matter how much you have attempted to distract yourself with last-minute work projects, batch cooking and choosing baby names, the prospect of the birth is never far from expectant mothers' minds.

Birth is an unpredictable process at the best of times, but when you are carrying twins it is at least doubly so. You will probably know the statistics already: your babies are more likely to be born prematurely, will weigh less (the average birth weight of a twin baby is 5 lb 5 oz, whereas the average birth weight of a single baby is 7 lb 5 oz) and have a higher chance of spending time in a special care unit than a single baby. On the plus side, they're unlikely to be overdue.

Don't forget that behind those figures lies huge variation. Many twins are born at or beyond the 37 weeks considered 'term' for all babies, and at comparable weights to single babies. There are plenty of examples in this chapter of babies born well beyond 37 weeks, including one set of twins who were born naturally on their 40-week due date. When parents of twins are asked when their babies were born, nearly all will give their answer in days as well as weeks. The extra risks associated with a twin pregnancy help to reinforce just how important each day in the womb is for the development of your babies – and no one appreciates this more than the mummies carrying this precious double cargo. This explains the twins' 'birth ages' included in many of the parents' quotes in this chapter.

Whilst it is a common scenario, don't assume that your babies will be premature, tiny and delivered by an emergency caesarean section. About 40 per cent of twins are born naturally (vaginally), and if you don't go into premature labour then elective caesareans provide a planned environment for the birth of your babies.

Best of all, don't assume anything. Your babies will come either when they and your body decides or, in more cases than with single babies, when your doctor advises that delivery is necessary for your or your babies' safety. Although this chapter will give you a useful picture of how labour and birth can pan out, your experience will be different. No two labours are the same, just as everyone's birth story is unique.

Planning your birth

Planning your twins' birth is an important and valuable exercise, but the chances are that reality will deviate – sometimes slightly and sometimes significantly – from your ideal birth. However, setting down your preferences for birth allows you to think through your contingency plans and it is a useful way of exploring all the likely scenarios before the big day.

Establish the following information from your hospital as a useful starting point:

▶ **Who will be present at your birth?** The short answer is usually quite a few people: at least one obstetrician, an anaesthetist, two midwives, a baby doctor for each baby, some students and other people whose identities you never discover. Even a vaginal birth involves most of these people on standby and may take place in the glare of an operating theatre.

▶ **Where might the birth take place?** Many hospitals don't allow twins to be born in their birthing suites and prefer the births to take place in an operating theatre. It is helpful to know this in advance.

▶ **What advice will be given about the birth?** If you are carrying twins, and especially if they share a placenta, your birth is considered higher risk and some hospitals will have a certain protocol, such as encouraging induction by a certain time, or an early elective caesarean. Birth procedures for identical twins vary enormously from hospital to hospital. Don't hesitate to quiz your consultant if you feel that this is not the birth you want or you do not understand the rationale behind it. You are entitled to do this and to negotiate details – or even refuse the advice.

▶ **What will happen if your babies are born early?** You may find it useful to visit their hospital's special care baby unit or neonatal intensive care ward before birth in order to prepare yourselves for the possibility of prematurity.

> 66 Touring the hospital was useful in demystifying the place. From my point of view I was going through this tectonic life shift, but for the hospital it was what they do every day. It was good to see it as a normal workplace. 99
>
> *Alicia, mum to Penny and Abe, six months*

When circumstances cause an elective C-section to be offered, some women feel relieved that one of the many uncertainties of carrying twins has been removed and are happy that they can plan for their arrival in this manner. Others feel disappointed or anxious, a feeling often made worse by the reaction of friends and family, which sometimes adds to the impression that to have a C-section is to somehow have crashed into the first hurdle of motherhood. However, as you will read, thousands of women find their elective C-section to be a calm and joyful experience, their babies are not damaged by being born 'too early' or without labour, and, provided you follow medical advice, recovery from surgery is usually straightforward.

‘‘ We resisted all attempts to book in a C-section. The consultant said to us that if we had our preferred choice of a natural birth we could end up with 'dead babies' — is that what we wanted? We were so shocked no one said anything. In fact we asked her to repeat herself. We had seen all the test results and knew the babies were fine so couldn't understand this attitude. We felt that we had all the information and that nothing was wrong, so wanted to carry on and try for a natural birth. It was shocking, even surreal and unnecessarily stressful. ’’

Ming, dad to Joseph and Alfred, two, born naturally at 39 weeks + three days

‘‘ My two previous pregnancies had been uncomplicated and I was determined to let labour start naturally. I really did not want to be induced because I felt it would lead to other interventions.

I met with consultants in the hospital, but I could see that I was getting nowhere.

At 38 weeks, a meeting was arranged with the hospital's midwife supervisor and a matron who was also an experienced midwife. I explained what I wanted and they went through the risks. I knew that my babies were head down, I didn't have high blood pressure and I wasn't overweight so I knew I could do it — I may not have been so brave if they'd been my first babies.

My advice is that you need to arm yourself with research. Have a realistic birth plan but start with what you want. Ask for the most experienced midwives the hospital has got. I found that unless you are really pushy the birth that you want is just not going to happen. 🙶

Susanne, mum to Delphie and Isadora, 22 months, born at 39 weeks + three days, weighing 7 lb 10 oz and 6 lb 13 oz respectively; Ana-Marie, six; and Nicolas, five

Your birth plan may not even be read or applicable when it is time for your twins to be born, but in compiling it, you and your partner will be clearer about your wishes and fears, which will allow you to ask better-informed questions as your care unfolds. It is fair to say that, for justifiable reasons, many – but by no means all – obstetricians are very cautious about the birth of twins and it can feel to some parents that they are happier to promote an elective C-section rather than risk complications, even if there is no evidence that complications are likely to arise.

It can feel difficult to challenge medical advice, particularly if it is presented in a way that suggests that to ignore the recommendation would put your babies at risk. Often there are good reasons behind the advice, but it is your right to question opinions with which you disagree and to ask for evidence to back up your consultant's recommendations. You can ask to deal with a more experienced obstetrician if necessary and should certainly ask for very experienced midwives to be present at your birth.

But however much we want to, birth is something that we can't control. In the end, a successful birth might be judged simply as the safe delivery of your babies and the good health of the mother.

Labour

Unlike some of the more obscure medical terminology, this word hits it on the nose. Labour. During which you will work extremely hard, but for the purpose and ultimate reward of, hopefully, two healthy babies. Knowing how the onset of labour could feel is important for soon-to-be mothers of twins, as you are more likely to experience labour at an unexpected time. Your womb will be stretched and expanded far more than it is anticipating, which can trigger a premature labour. You may experience problems in your own health, such as signs of pre-eclampsia or bleeding or your waters breaking early, which may necessitate early delivery, either through induced labour or a C-section.

Premature labour

If you experience any of the following symptoms, phone your maternity ward immediately for further guidance. Don't assume it can't be labour because your pregnancy is not far enough advanced. Things can move very quickly with premature twins, so if you have any concerns at all, phone the hospital.

Seek medical advice if:

► You have a low, heavy, period-like pain in your tummy or lower back, especially if it comes and goes

► There are mucus discharges or there is bleeding from your vagina

► Your waters break or there is a leakage of clear fluid from the vagina

► You have regular contractions

See the next chapter for more details on prematurity.

66 Premature labour happens to a bigger percentage of women with twins, but every woman should be prepared that they may go into labour at any time. In twins the uterus gets more stretched, which is why the uterus thinks it's nine months when it's eight months or less. Even a labour that ends in a caesarean is not pointless from the mother's or babies' point of view; labour is maturing for the baby so even if it ends in a caesarean it has done them some good and given them some maturity. 99

Dr Susan Bewley, professor of complex obstetrics,
King's College London

66 I woke up at 2 a.m. and could feel some wetness. I got up and went to the loo and it just didn't stop, which is when I realised my waters had broken. I felt fine, I had a shower and hadn't had any contractions – except some that felt like a bit of period pain. The hospital told us to come straight in and within half an hour of arriving I started having a few light contractions, which very quickly started coming very close together. After a couple of climbing-the-wall contractions and about an hour after arriving at the hospital I told the midwife that I needed a poo. She checked and I was fully dilated. I was ready to push. Lola was born first and Franklin followed 14 minutes later. I don't think anything could have prepared me for the birth – I just didn't think it would happen to me. I never thought that I'd have the babies when I went in – I assumed they'd try to stave off labour as much as possible. It felt a bit weird. 99

Sally, mum to Lola and Franklin, six months. They were born
at 33 weeks, weighing 3 lb 13 oz and 3 lb 14 oz respectively

The early stage of labour

Every mother dreads first knowing of her labour when she is standing in a supermarket surrounded by a pool of amniotic fluid. Fortunately, for many women, labour begins with a very mild sensation of period pain, an uncomfortable feeling low in the tummy and a 'show' – a plug of bloody mucus that has come away from the cervix. Although your waters can break at any stage in this process, it commonly happens in the later stages of labour and it is not unusual for a mother's waters to have to be broken by a midwife.

Don't be confused by Braxton Hicks contractions, which you will probably experience earlier in your pregnancy. Unlike the real thing, Braxton Hicks contractions are painless and irregular tightening sensations from the uterus, and are not an indicator that labour has begun. You can continue as normal during these low-level contractions.

At this point, your body is preparing itself to give birth by softening, lengthening and thinning your cervix, the neck of your womb. When soft and thin enough, it will begin to open or dilate. This can take upwards of 12 hours or it may happen quite quickly, especially if this is not your first pregnancy. Your contractions will be cranking up, but will probably still be quite short and be widely spaced. Be warned: if you can talk through the contractions then you are still in the foothills of this particular expedition.

Your cervix will start to dilate, but only by a few centimetres. Don't forget that your contractions are pushing your babies down and preparing your cervix to let them out, as well as readying your twins for the outside world – they're all for a purpose! As your contractions increase in frequency and intensity, they will feel like waves of pain washing over you. For a few seconds it is unbearable, and you can't speak or think about anything else, then the wave breaks and you can function normally for a minute or two until the contractions start again.

Tips for managing contractions:

▶ Keep moving around or changing position

▶ If you find a comfy place, such as a warm bath, stay in it

▶ Keep your fluids up by drinking water or sports/energy drinks

▶ Remind yourself that each contraction is bringing you closer to your babies

▶ Use relaxation CDs, breathing or hypnobirthing techniques

▶ Counting during the painful part of a contraction can remind you that it will end ('One elephant, two elephants… ')

▶ Time how often your contractions come. It's good to keep tabs on your progress and it gives your partner something to do. Don't obsess over the timings, however

▶ Use TENS (transcutaneous electrical nerve stimulation) machines. Available for hire, TENS machines are taped on to your back and connected by wires to a small battery-powered stimulator. It is thought that they encourage the body to produce more of its own natural painkillers. While it is best not to place too much reliance on this option, these machines can provide some pain relief in the early part of labour.

When your contractions last 30–60 seconds and occur every five minutes, call your midwife for guidance. It is probably time to head to the hospital if you are not there already.

Active labour – or not

In mothers carrying twins, 'active labour' can be a bit of a misnomer. One of the obsessions of the labour ward is tracking the heartbeats of your babies. In practice this means strapping two lots of monitoring equipment across your vast girth and then checking to make sure the information has come through properly. All too often, one or both sets slip, or both sets pick up the same heartbeat, occasionally causing unnecessary panic. The result is that you can feel pinned to the bed when what you want to be doing is walking around, squatting, pounding your fists against a wall – or anything else that eases the pain. In short, you are often anything but active at this point.

You will receive a lot of interruptions and attention from a fairly large medical team and it is at this point that serious pain relief is in the offing if you need it. This will take the form of gas and air, epidurals (where painkillers are passed to the small of your back via a fine tube) or various pain-relief drugs. Epidurals once knocked out the whole of the bottom half of your body, but are now more subtle in their effect and can allow you to retain some mobility and feeling. Sometimes, after a flurry of activity, the momentum goes out of labour and no progress is made at all. In this instance, you may be given a pessary (a medical device inserted into the vagina) or put on a drip to induce stronger contractions again and speed up dilation, as this can be an exhausting process for both you and the babies.

Your midwife will be checking how dilated your cervix is becoming. By the time you are 7 cm–8 cm dilated, you will be near the end of this first stage of labour.

Transition

You are now chipping away at the coalface of the birth process. At the point just before the 'second' stage of labour, it is not uncommon to feel nauseous or to vomit. Grit your teeth, shriek and demand pain relief if you need it – this 'transition' stage is really hard, painful work, which could last anything between a few minutes to a few hours. Hopefully sooner rather than later, you will receive the happy news that you have hit the jackpot and are ready to push. You may want to push well before this 10 cm dilation stage, but to do so could cause damage to your cervix.

> 66 I was induced using a pessary which brought on really strong contractions, but I didn't dilate at all. Jed was lying with his back to my back, which triggered terrible back pain. Because I wasn't dilated they refused to give me an epidural. After a few hours of total agony they stopped trying with the pessary, gave me pethidine [a painkiller] and let me sleep. They then tried to break my waters, which wasn't successful and after that I told them I wasn't having anything else done without an epidural. I was given an epidural and a drip to induce labour and dozed from about 9 p.m. to 7 a.m. It seems bizarre to be able to sleep through the contractions and get to full dilation, but that's what happened. 99
>
> *Mercedes, mum to Jed and Millie, two weeks, born at 38 weeks + two days, weighing 6 lb and 5 lb 8 oz respectively*

Vaginal birth

Many women find that it is around this stage that their veneer of twenty-first-century sophistication disappears, to be replaced by a primordial cavewoman in an NHS gown. This is perhaps the only time in your life when all normal etiquette ceases to apply and you behave in a way that is completely out of character. You may swear at a doctor or your partner, howl like a dog, groan like a donkey – whatever it takes to get your babies safely into the outside world. The best of it is that you won't care, or possibly even notice.

You will experience a very strong urge to push and your midwife will guide you to maximise each push. As a general guide, giving birth feels like you are doing a poo the size of a watermelon and all your pushing is concentrated in that area. You may well pass some poo in the process, which is completely normal and something midwives are used to dealing with, and discreetly removing.

When the first baby's head is almost out, you will be asked to stop or give a more gentle push to protect the skin of the perineum (the area of skin between your vagina and anus).

Your first baby is out, but the focus will be on the safe delivery of your second baby. Depending on the circumstances, Baby One may be given to you to suckle to encourage more oxytocin, often called the 'love hormone', which will also help bring on contractions for Baby Two. Sometimes, though, Baby One will be whisked away to be checked and cleaned up while you concentrate on the next one. Some mothers report that they rested until they felt the urge to push; others that they felt tremendous pressure from medical staff to push straight away. Generally, doctors want to monitor the second baby to make sure it is lined up properly to go down the birth canal. They don't like a period of more than an hour to elapse between the birth of the two babies as there is evidence that risks to the unborn twin increase after this point.

Once the babies have been born, there is still some work to do as the placentas, which have been sustaining your babies in the womb and are now redundant, need to be delivered, too. Some women say they barely noticed this part with all the fuss and drama of their twins' arrival, while others were surprised that they were required to do more pushing, even after the babies were out.

> 66 Usually, Baby One is born, breathes and cries. After at least a minute or two, the cord is clamped and then the next baby presents at the cervix and will be born, followed by both placentas. We tend to put one clip on the first cord, then two clips on the second to identify them. One worry is that with the sudden decompression of the uterus, contractions will lead to placenta(s) separating. If this happens you can get Baby One, followed by placenta one, then Baby Two and placenta two. If the placenta starts separating then Baby Two can be in trouble. This is one of the reasons people are anxious about a long gap. 99
>
> *Dr Susan Bewley, professor of complex obstetrics,*
> *King's College London*

In normal circumstances, mothers of twins will be given a routine injection of Syntocinon after the birth, which speeds up the delivery of the placentas and reduces the chance of heavy bleeding. Thanks to your two passengers, you have a greater blood flow to the uterus and bigger 'raw area' where the placentas sat – and therefore a higher risk of significant blood loss.

If you have experienced rips or tears in your perineum, you will be stitched up in the delivery room. This can result in yet more undignified positioning and pain. Some women are beyond caring; for others it is an unexpected and uncomfortable start to motherhood.

> 66 Contractions started in the early hours of their 40-week due date and I was worried I'd have them in the taxi to the hospital.

A room was waiting for us and there were about ten million people in there. No one had had time to read my birth plan and, although I wasn't conscious of this at the time, with hindsight I was not in control. Maui was born within 15 minutes of arriving at hospital. In my birth plan I'd said I didn't want the cord to be cut until it had stopped pulsating, but they did it straight away. Everyone was shouting at me to push. There was no time to think or for my feelings to be expressed. Loki was born 15 minutes later. I feel blessed that I carried them to term and they were healthy, but there is a lot of panic about twins among consultants. Sometimes women do know what to do with their bodies and I don't think that should be discredited. 🙶

Adwoa, mum to Ti-Jean, six; Maui and Loki, two, born at 40 weeks, weighing 7 lb 8 oz and 6 lb 3 oz respectively

🙷 The midwife had given me her mobile number so she met me at the hospital. I had really wanted a water birth and they'd told me I could do it for the first twin, but that the second might change position, so I'd need to get out of the water for the second birth. I had also said I didn't want a consultant in the room – we were in a hospital, so if they were needed they could be called. The only people present at the birth were the hospital's midwife supervisor and two senior midwives as well as my husband. The babies were born just as planned. I felt overjoyed – the birth was just as it should have been. 🙶

Susanne, mum to Delphie and Isadora, 22 months, born at 39 weeks + three days, weighing 7 lb 10 oz and 6 lb 13 oz respectively; Ana-Marie, six; and Nicolas, five

Forceps and ventouse deliveries

Sometimes women have what is called an 'assisted birth', when one or both of their babies are delivered vaginally with the help of forceps (which look like big metal tongs) or ventouse (a big vacuum hose). This can happen because a baby is in an awkward position, a mother is too tired to push or there are concerns about a baby's heartbeat.

Both procedures involve an episiotomy (small cut to the vaginal wall) which is done under local anaesthetic if an epidural hasn't already been given. Forceps are curved to fit round a baby's head and, as you push, an obstetrician pulls to help deliver the baby.

Ventouse works using suction and is attached to a baby's head using a cup. Again, an obstetrician will pull to coincide with a mother's pushes and contractions to deliver the baby. Babies delivered by ventouse will have a small swelling on their heads (called a chignon) and there is often bruising, both of which should disappear quite quickly after birth. Forceps-delivered babies can also have bruising or small cuts to their faces or heads.

Assisted deliveries increase the risk of vaginal and anal tears to the mother and there is also a greater likelihood of suffering either anal or urinary incontinence.

Birth by caesarean section

Having read all that, some women might be forgiven for thinking that delivery by C-section is an 'easier' option, but don't be fooled. As your doctors will have explained, a C-section is major surgery, which, in bypassing labour, also deprives your babies of the usual natural processes which mature them, clear their lungs and prepare them for the outside world. The risks to you, the mother, are also higher than a vaginal birth, with an increased chance of infection, blood clots and adhesions (where scar tissue makes organs in your tummy stick to each other). No one should feel bad about having a C-section if it is needed, and circumstances may dictate that this is the best option for you and your babies, but it is important to be aware of both the benefits and risks of the procedure.

There are two types of C-section. An elective caesarean, which takes place before labour has started and the date of which is planned with your consultant. An emergency C-section, which may happen before or during labour, when an unexpected complication has arisen and the babies need to be delivered quickly.

Reasons why babies need to be born via C-section include:

▶ The babies' position – If the first baby is lying sideways (transverse) or breech (feet or bottom first)

▶ Your condition – You may have a low-lying placenta which is blocking the babies' exit route or you may suffer from an illness which makes a C-section advisable

▶ The twins sharing a placenta – The hospital may consider it safer to deliver identical twins in this way because of the theoretical risk of a blood transfusion between the twins, called an inter-twin transfusion, during labour

▶ An emergency arising during labour – Such as one or both of the babies becoming distressed in the womb, so that they cannot be delivered through the vagina

▶ The labour failing to progress and both the mother and the babies are exhausted

Beforehand you will have signed a consent form that details the risks of a C-section to both you and the babies, as well as taken medication to reduce the acid in your stomach. You will not have eaten for 12 hours prior to your C-section. Antibiotics will have been offered as a way of preventing post-operative infection.

A C-section takes place in an operating theatre with a large cast of participants: there will be at least two obstetricians, an anaesthetist and anaesthetic assistant, two midwives, two paediatricians, a 'scrub nurse', a specialist trained to work in an operating theatre, and runner, who supports the staff in theatre, plus the likelihood of a few students.

The surgery itself is likely to take less than 45 minutes. The process begins with the anaesthetist giving you an epidural, which is fed into your lower back via a fine tube. You will also have a tube (catheter) inserted into your bladder to empty it, and a drip put into your arm or hand so you can have extra pain relief or fluids if necessary.

A screen will be put across your tummy so you don't see what's going on. The obstetrician will make a small cut of about 20 cm in your lower abdomen, followed by a second cut in your womb, from where the babies are easily extracted within minutes. Warning: some partners are shocked by the amount of blood and gore they see when they peek over the screen to catch a first glimpse of the babies. Some mothers say they regret not witnessing the moment when their babies entered the world. You can ask hospital staff to lower the screen or to adjust the mirror (if one is attached to the theatre light) if you prefer to witness it all. Your bump will hide the wound, but you will see the babies as soon as they emerge.

You shouldn't experience any pain during this process; many women describe the sensation as like someone rummaging in a handbag or doing the washing-up in their tummy.

66 I said to the anaesthetist that I was really scared about the point at which they started cutting and asked her to warn me. She told me they'd already started. I felt nothing at that stage, but did feel them rummaging about to get the babies which felt weird, but not painful. 99

Alicia, mum to Penny and Abe, six months, born at 35 weeks, weighing 5 lb 4 oz and 5 lb 6 oz respectively

> 66 It was a bit like a magic act – because of the screen it didn't look like the lower half belonged to my partner. I looked over and I could see everything, her stomach wall and both the babies inside. It was a bit like those magazines you buy for children where they assemble the human body. It was surreal to see a human cut open like that and still be alive and talking to you from above the screen. 99
>
> *Darren, dad to Mattie and Evie, ten; and Eliza, three*

The placenta(s) will be delivered and the wounds will then be sewn up using dissolvable stitches or staples, and you will be moved with the babies fairly swiftly into a recovery room.

As this is major surgery, you have an increased risk of blood clots so will have to wear support stockings and may have to inject yourself (into your tummy or thigh) with blood-thinning drugs for a week or so after your discharge from hospital. Getting up and about as soon as you are able helps recovery, and reduces the risk of blood clots and chest infections. It may seem harsh, but you will be encouraged to get out of bed quite quickly once the epidural wears off.

> 66 We were told to arrive from 7 a.m. and I knew it was first come, first served. Just as we were about to leave, our dog did a massive poo on the doormat. It was like a protest. By the time we'd cleared it up we didn't get to the hospital until 7.10 a.m. and were last in the queue! The birth itself happened very quickly – from having the epidural to being taken to the recovery room post-birth took about 40 minutes. I remember

them not showing me the first baby because they were obviously thinking about the next one and I was thinking that I couldn't hear her cry, then the second one was shown to me and I could hear the first one crying. 〞

Alison, mum to Sylvie and Mila, 12 months, born at 38 weeks, weighing 6 lb and 6 lb 4 oz respectively

❝ I'd really been dreading having a C-section and was trying to avoid it, but actually it was quite a pleasant experience. We were upstairs in a room with windows with sunshine pouring in and it felt rather wonderful. The staff all seemed very calm and capable, and it was very positive. 〞

Mercedes, mum to Jed and Millie, two weeks, born at 38 weeks + two days, weighing 6 lb and 5 lb 8 oz respectively

Tips for a C-section birth:

▶ You will have major surgery, and you will need – and receive – major pain relief. Don't be a heroine – take all your medication and ask for more if you are in pain. Don't wait until it is excruciating before making a fuss as you may need more and stronger doses than if you take it regularly.

▶ Although it may be the last thing you want to do, try to move about as much as you can, and as quickly as you can, as this will really help your recovery.

▶ Getting out of bed for the first time will be really hard and you may feel as if your insides are about to fall out. They aren't.

▶ You may shake quite violently or vomit in the hours after your C-section.

▶ Invest in some large pants (the ones that finish under your boobs) a few sizes bigger than your actual size. You won't want anything that rubs against your wound. Get lots of disposables so you can throw away pants that get very bloody.

▶ You will still bleed as if you had given birth vaginally, so you will need plenty of thick sanitary pads. You could also try sticking a sanitary pad to the front part of your pants to shield your C-section wound.

▶ Constipation is a common problem after a C-section. Bring prunes or a good fibre source into hospital to avoid this.

▶ Nighties are more practical than pyjamas at this stage as they are easier to get on. You'll need more than one as they, too, are likely to get stained or bloody.

▶ Use a pillow to press against your wound in order to get out of bed more comfortably.

▶ Bring cartons of drinks with straws that you can drink without having to move too much.

Recovery in hospital

The best thing about reaching the postnatal ward is that it means you are only one step away from going home. And, after the first night, you may well be pleading with doctors to speed up your discharge. With some honourable exceptions, postnatal wards are notoriously overstretched and are not geared up to dealing with mothers with two babies – particularly immobile ones recovering from a C-section.

The postnatal wards are generally noisy and busy. Unexpected visitors will regularly appear at your bedside to do a hearing test on the babies or to give you a free nappy sample or carry out some other unexpected test or check. Someone will pop up and ask you if you have considered what contraceptive device you'll be using when you return home. Amid all this, you will be attempting to get your babies to latch on or stop crying, usually unaided as partners are not allowed to stay overnight on the ward. In short, the chances of losing it within a few hours of hitting the ward are high. On the plus side, a weeping mum accompanied by the stereo wails of her babies can be very effective for focusing the staff's minds on finding you a separate room where you can get some support from a partner or relative.

66 On the second day my catheter came out and I was told I could get on my feet. It was really hard to move and to walk to the toilet. Art didn't want to latch on and I was crying. The hospital allowed partners to visit in the morning but everyone else had to come at 3 p.m. I wanted my mum to come in early to help me but the hospital wouldn't let her. It was the weekend and I remember pressing the button because I needed help with feeding and the midwife came and said "What do you want me to do? I'm so busy!" At that point I discharged myself. 99

Pornthida, mum to Art and Enda, five months, born at 37 weeks, weighing 6 lb 8 oz and 7 lb 2 oz respectively

66 It was really hard in the hospital. I was taken to the shower and then just left there. I had blood pouring out of me. What could I do? I couldn't even get my clothes back on. I just wanted to get out of the hospital. But within about ten days I felt pretty good. It really wasn't as bad as I thought it was going to be. It is a bit weird because you can't see your scar when you take off your dressing because your stomach is in the way. I didn't want to look at it. 99

Alison, mum to Sylvie and Mila, 12 months, born at 38 weeks, weighing 6 lb and 6 lb 4 oz respectively

You may feel that a rather unflattering picture is emerging of NHS postnatal care for mothers of twins. It should, of course, be stressed that there are many dedicated, expert midwives in our hospitals who will provide you and your twins with fantastic care. Nearly every mother can name a midwife to whom no amount of gratitude will adequately express the enormity of their help in delivering their twins safely. Hopefully this book will help you to recognise those wonderful midwives and have the confidence to ask more of those who fall short of that gold standard.

Above all, remember that if you want help or advice or simply need reassurance about what you should be doing, ask for it – forcefully. Or get your partner or visiting friend to do so. You are a new mum of twins, who could be more important?

Home birth

It takes an extremely brave woman to have twins at home, but it does happen. The NHS will not support a home birth for twins because the risks are considered too great, so as a result they are rare. However, every year a small number of women take matters into their own hands by employing an independent midwife to oversee their care. As discussed in Chapter 5, an independent midwife is a fully qualified and highly experienced midwife who has chosen to work outside the NHS. A minimum of three midwives are present at a home birth for twins (one for each baby and one for the mother) and the lead midwife will liaise with the NHS over the progress of the birth, in case it is necessary to go into hospital.

Postnatal care would be carried out either by the mother's independent midwife or by an NHS community midwife and, later, a health visitor.

    ❝ I had a very traumatic experience at the birth of my first son. I had so many interventions 'just in case' and every part of it was a fight. As a result, I didn't want any scans with my second pregnancy and had a home birth planned. However, two months before the baby was due, I discovered I was expecting twins. At which point my husband and I panicked because we thought it was going to be another experience like our first birth.

    We were really lucky to find an independent midwife who was very experienced and confident in dealing with a twin birth, and at last we started to meet people who were positive and trusted our intuition. We don't come from the category of people who can consider employing an independent midwife, but we felt this was something we were prepared to go into debt over, if we had to. We knew all the risks and were realistic about things and would have gone into hospital if there had been any concerns at the birth.

    My waters broke just after 8 a.m. and then labour started. I had agreed to have a student midwife present and Annabel also brought two other midwives. They were so encouraging and reassuring.

    At about noon I got into the birthing pool and Helena was born first at 3 p.m. It was amazing and I held her in my arms for a minute, but very quickly felt a contraction so I passed her to Annabel. I thought I was birthing the placenta, because it felt so soft and I hardly had to push, but it was the second baby who shot out like a bullet. There were only four minutes between them! Neither of them cried and it felt such a normal and quiet event; something to celebrate, but nothing to be afraid of.

    Everyone has their own perspective on birth, but for my husband and I it was a healing and empowering experience which put me on a high for months. I feel so grateful. ❞

Monika, mum to Matilda and Helena, 15 months, born at 38 weeks + three days, weighing 6 lb 2 oz and 6 lb 8 oz respectively; and Filip, five

How birth works – your babies' perspective

As you are puffing and groaning through labour, you probably won't have much time to marvel at nature's ingenious system of propelling your babies into the world. You may well be wishing labour had never evolved at all. But it really all is for a purpose and even if your labour ends with a C-section, your hard work during labour is helping your babies undergo a tremendous transformation – from passengers in your womb to separate beings capable of breathing by themselves.

Cocooned in amniotic fluid in your womb, your twins rely on your placenta(s) to receive their nourishment and oxygen, as well as to expel their waste. Their lungs are filled with fluid.

As labour kicks in and contractions become more frequent, your cervix dilates and your body prepares to push and squeeze your babies down through the birth canal. The babies experience slight stress from the contractions, as their blood supply is temporarily cut off with each contraction and this leads to their lungs being emptied of fluid. This is the body's way of preparing the babies for the jolt of the next and dramatic stage of their development. Very soon they will have to take their first breath of air and continue breathing on their own – being alert and full of adrenaline helps them to achieve this.

As the first baby comes through the birth canal, its ribs are squeezed, creating more pressure to clear fluid from its lungs. The release of this pressure as the baby is born causes air to be drawn into the lungs, enabling its first, important breath. In the first few minutes after birth, blood from the placenta moves into the blood vessels of the baby's lungs. Previously, in utero, oxygen was extracted from the placenta. Babies have a special blood that can sustain them on low oxygen levels, which is why they are blue before and immediately after birth. After the first breaths of air through the lungs, the babies gradually turn a more normal colour as their oxygen levels increase. Parents understandably panic at the prospect of the umbilical cord becoming wrapped round the babies' necks, but this is a relatively common occurrence: one in 100 babies is born with the cord around its neck and is not 'strangled'.

As discussed in Chapter 2, your babies' sense of smell began to develop in the womb, and they are already familiar with your scent, which is what they are both drawn to immediately after birth, as well as the attractive smell of your breast milk.

At birth, each baby's central nervous system is stimulated. The baby's lungs expand to oxygenate its own blood, and the kidneys and liver take over from the placenta to filter the blood.

While many twin births are by caesarean section, this does not necessarily mean that you will avoid labour, or at least the first stages of labour. After a non-labour caesarean, most babies will breathe and clear their lung fluid, but there are higher chances of breathing difficulties and help being required as the babies have to work a bit harder to clear the fluid. Although the mother works really hard in labour, so do your babies – and the developmental steps that they take as they emerge into the world are truly amazing.

Coming to terms with your birth

Giving birth is a rite of passage from which you may feel yourself emerge as a different person. It is an experience that can never be fully prepared for and, sometimes, it leaves you full of questions, anxiety and even trauma. If you feel overwhelmed by your birth experience – or are angry, confused or upset at what you went through – it is important to try to get some answers while you are still in hospital as your notes and the people who cared for you are readily available.

It is good practice for the doctor who delivered your babies to visit you after the birth, but that doesn't always happen. You can ask to speak to them or you can ask a midwife to explain the birth using your hospital notes, which should detail the reasons behind each medical decision. Try to deal with your questions while they are fresh in your mind and there are people around to answer them. This should help you understand and come to terms with your experience.

66 I had a really long labour that stopped and started and had to be induced, but once my waters were broken things speeded up. Everything seemed to be going well until Mia's heart rate went really high. Everyone was telling me to push, but I didn't feel the urge to push at all and couldn't do it so I had an emergency C-section to get her out. Mia had to be resuscitated, although we didn't find that out for four days. Afterwards I felt more disappointed that the birth hadn't gone the way I'd been planning than excited about the fact the babies were here. Mia had been taken straight to the neonatal intensive-care unit, but Willow was fine. They gave my partner a photo of Mia in NICU and it was a really, really distressing photo, which made me worry even more. We kept asking what had happened and why Mia was in NICU, but the nurses told us that the doctors were busy or that an emergency had come up. In the end, I had to get a nurse to wheel me round to the NICU so that I could catch the doctors on their rounds at 9 a.m. and finally I got some answers. I felt quite low those first few days, but felt I couldn't admit it as I'd be judged for it. Now that a bit of time has passed, I have got this overwhelming urge that I need to have another baby and do it 'right' this time, because I feel I'm not as much of a mum as anyone else because I haven't done it properly. 99

Emily, mum to Willow and Mia, six weeks, born at 36 weeks + six days, weighing 5 lb 8 oz each

66 Watching women give birth over the past 40 years, since I was a student, I think it may be harder to be pregnant and give birth than ever before — there's more for women to juggle in their lives, there's less family and community support, there's so much more available and conflicting information, and there's more finger pointing of guilt and blame. You enter a state of uncertainty and loss of control. Perhaps that's why pregnancy is nine months long — so that women can get their head round the fact that, in some senses, they've lost control forever. It can be hard, or exhilarating, to embrace that. 99

Dr Susan Bewley, professor of complex obstetrics,
King's College London

Chapter 8

Premature Twins

This chapter more than any other is a reminder that the arrival of every pair of healthy twins should be celebrated as nothing less than a miracle. Because, despite the fact that nature regularly throws double pregnancies our way, women's bodies are not really designed to carry more than one baby at a time; the strain of doing so can result in complications, creating a far greater likelihood of premature arrivals.

A lot of the information in this chapter makes for difficult reading. As parents looking forward to the birth of twins, you hope for a safe delivery of good-sized, healthy babies. However, the fact is that half of all twins are born early, before 37 weeks. Six per cent of those, between 500–600 sets of twins a year, will arrive extremely early, between 28 and 31 weeks, and some even earlier.

It is often not possible to predict which pregnancies will end early and many women prefer not to think about it on the basis that it may never happen. For others, gaining a small insight into life with premature babies may be helpful or reassuring, and although you can never fully prepare for seeing your own babies in an incubator, understanding what could happen may lessen your anxiety.

Why are twins born early?

Some factors, such as problems with the mother's health or the development of one or both of the babies in the womb, may provide a clue that your twins are likely to be delivered early. Other factors can include infections, the uterus becoming prematurely stretched, the placenta(s) failing to sustain the babies and the mother's lifestyle (smoking and taking recreational drugs, for example). However, the reason behind many premature arrivals is never known and, usually, could not have been prevented.

The most common reasons for preterm births:

▶ **Pre-eclampsia** – A condition that can threaten both the babies and mother if undetected. It is most likely to be picked up by high blood pressure and protein in the mother's urine.

▶ **Placenta praevia** – Where the placenta is lying low and blocking the babies' way out. This is usually accompanied by vaginal bleeding.

▶ **Gestational diabetes** – When some women have such high levels of blood glucose during pregnancy that their body is unable to produce enough insulin to absorb it all.

▶ **Intrauterine growth restriction** – Where one twin is not getting enough sustenance from the placenta and its growth is affected. The babies will be closely monitored for as long as possible, until their safety means delivery is unavoidable – if the doctors feel that the placenta is no longer working.

▶ **Twin-to-twin transfusion syndrome** – This results in an uneven blood distribution from one twin to the other in the womb and affects 10–15 per cent of babies sharing a placenta. This will be monitored very closely and can result in a preterm birth. This condition is potentially fatal.

> 66 I was diagnosed with placenta praevia and bled constantly –
> like a period – pretty much throughout my pregnancy. At 23
> weeks and six days I was admitted and told I would stay there
> until the babies arrived.
>
> It was like a ticking time bomb. They wouldn't tell me that
> I would be OK because they didn't know and they wouldn't
> tell me the babies would be OK, because they didn't know
> that either.
>
> Every time I bled – which was about three times a week
> and they were heavy bleeds – all the monitors were brought
> back in and I lay there shaking thinking, 'Is this it?' It wasn't
> and then we'd go through it all again. 99
>
> *Anna, mum to Mia and Sam, seven months, born at 30*
> *weeks, weighing 3 lb and 3.1 lb respectively; Harry, ten;*
> *and Olivia, 13*

What problems will premature twins face?

Every day spent in the womb is crucial to the development of your twins, which is why doctors will do all they can to stave off an early delivery unless the mother or babies' health is threatened. The problems premature babies face very much depend on how early they are and it is impossible to predict the long-term implications because each baby is different.

Many premature babies have breathing difficulties, because the lungs are one of the last organs to develop before birth, which is why you will receive a course of steroid injections to help your twins' lungs mature if they need to be delivered at 34 weeks or younger. The injection would be given the day before the birth as it takes 24 hours to work.

Statistics tell us that twins are more likely than single babies to develop cerebral palsy, a general term for a number of neurological conditions that affect movement and coordination, because two key risk factors are premature birth and low birth weight.

Prematurity brings with it increased chances of deafness, asthma, sight problems, developmental delays and other complications. But, incredibly, some babies born very early can and do make a full recovery, catching up with their peers over several years.

Try not to look too far ahead if your twins are born early. It is very frightening to see your babies looking so tiny and spindly, and dependent on intensive care, but many do defy the odds.

Life with babies in special care

The unexpected or rapid arrival of your babies may mean you don't have a chance to cuddle or even see them before the doctors whisk them away to a neonatal intensive care unit or special care baby unit. Everything is likely to have happened quickly and, with so much focus on the babies, you may be feeling shocked, lost and scared. Your own health may be poor and may prevent you from seeing your babies. At times it may feel like you are bystanders with no control over what happens to your new arrivals.

Once the initial urgency at their birth has calmed down, you will be able to visit them in the neonatal unit. To begin with, if your babies are very tiny, it may not be possible to hold them, but you will be encouraged to spend time with them, to touch them if appropriate, and to talk to them, to reinforce your comforting presence. Nurses will involve you in the babies' care as much as possible and, as discussed in Chapter 10, you will be encouraged to express colostrum and milk to be given to your twins.

As your babies progress, you will be able to have skin-to-skin contact or 'kangaroo care' where you tuck one baby at a time chest-to-chest against your skin.

" I was very apprehensive about visiting the neonatal unit – I think I was scared of what I was going to see. In fact, it calmed me to see babies of 24 or 25 weeks, which is what my unborn twins were at that stage. They were babies – just very little ones with some wires.

Despite that visit, nothing can prepare you for seeing your own babies in the neonatal unit. I was very apprehensive about going in and seeing them and found it very daunting because of the beeping of monitors. Even now if my husband forgets to put his seatbelt on quickly, it sets off an alarm in the car that reminds me of the monitors, which I can't cope with at all.

One night Mia had dirtied her incubator, so they put her in with Sam while they cleaned it. As soon as they were in there together all the monitors went quiet. Not a single beep went off. As soon as she was put back again they started.

The hardest thing was coming home without them. I sat in hospital for six weeks and saw so many people come in with their bumps and leave with their car seats. I felt cheated that I didn't do that. "

Anna, mum to Mia and Sam, seven months, born at 30 weeks, weighing 3 lb and 3.1 lb respectively; Harry, ten; and Olivia, 13

" The first time we saw them was about 12 hours after their birth. They were wrapped in foil with UV masks on. They were tiny, pink, shrivelly things. It was quite frightening. We both came out of the ward and said, 'That was really weird.' Part of you wonders – 'Is that really my baby?'

It feels like you are a part-time parent. You can feed them and change them and hold them, but there's not much else you can do. We tried to go out a few times because we knew we wouldn't get a chance when they came home, but it just felt wrong to have babies in special care and be sitting in the pub. "

Jayne, mum to Thomas and Holly, 11 months, born at 33 weeks, weighing 2 lb 15 oz and 2 lb 11 oz respectively

"I remember how loud the intensive care unit was. There were eight really big incubators all hooked up to lots of bits of equipment. There was a nurse assigned to each incubator and then a doctor between two. There seemed to be a lot of people. It was a slightly scary, stressful and emotional place, a bit like a weird sci-fi movie.

I felt like they weren't quite mine – like the medical staff had a higher claim over them than me. When they were very poorly I was OK about it, but when Rosa was moved to an open incubator and had nothing attached to her I still had to ask permission to pick her up, which I didn't understand."

Romany, mum to Rosa and Phoenix, five, born at 30 weeks + six days, weighing 3 lb 9 oz and 4 lb 8 oz respectively

As the parents of twins in special care, you have the additional worry of two babies, two sets of bleeping monitors and dividing your time and love between the incubators. It is quite normal to feel scared of holding such fragile-looking babies and sometimes bonding with your premature twins takes longer than you might be expecting. The strain and uncertainty of having tiny babies in special care is exhausting and for a while it may feel as if your life has shrunk to the neonatal unit, with everything else deemed irrelevant. Your day could involve spending eight to ten hours (or more) sitting by their incubators, which can be draining and difficult to manage if you have other children to care for, too.

> 66 We did feel pressured. The hospital wanted to know why one of us couldn't stay. We explained that every day we left the hospital crying, but we also had two other children who needed us. The twins didn't understand if we were there or not, but the girls did. 99
>
> *Clare, mum to Henley and Riley, 19 months; Lexi, three; and Kaysie, nine*

Your babies will stay in special care until they can feed and regulate their own temperature, and the staff are confident that their needs can be accommodated at home. As a general rule-of-thumb guide, premature babies usually stay in hospital until their original due date. However, this doesn't always happen in practice and if one or both babies are making good progress they can be discharged earlier.

With luck, you will find invaluable support and understanding among the parents you meet in the special care unit who are experiencing similar emotions. Lasting friendships are often forged as a result of this connection.

Leaving hospital

When you have babies in special care, not only do you leave hospital before them, but it is quite likely that one twin will be discharged before the other.

If possible, parents can 'room' with their babies in hospital for a night to prepare for looking after them alone at home, but this is not always the case.

> 66 It had never occurred to me that the boys would not be discharged together. We were given no warning – we came in on the Monday and were told Mohan was being discharged that day. After he had been discharged I expressed milk and sent it in with my husband the next day. I felt terrible that I had to choose between which baby to see. A bit later the nurse rang and said, 'Your son is here, when are you coming to see him?' What was I supposed to do? 99
>
> *Neela, mum to Mohan and Rohan, 23 months, born at 34 weeks, weighing 5 lb 4 oz each; and Asha, four*

All the usual anxieties about managing on your own at home are magnified with premature babies. Having experienced a high level of care over weeks or months, the prospect of having to cope without the safety net of the constant presence of highly skilled nurses is worrying for many parents. However, some parents feel that this is when their twin parenting really starts and find the experience of leaving hospital liberating and exciting – the chance to be a family at last.

> 66 Our son was ready to come home first. He had spent some time in intensive care, then special care and after two months he was ready to come home. Even though having prem twins is a very traumatic experience, we had become quite used to hospital life and other parents and staff had become our support network. So my first reaction was 'I don't want him home, I'm not ready'. Also the thought of having one child at home and the other in hospital was daunting.

I really was unprepared at home as I had not bought a thing because I did not want to tempt fate. So my husband and I spent one night in a room in hospital with my son to get used to having sole care and so I could still go through and see my daughter on the ward. The next morning we took Alexander home in a second-hand single pram that my mum had managed to get the day before.

The first night seemed relatively easy but it was strange not having the noise of all the hospital machines bleeping. Next morning I went straight to hospital with Alexander. I put him into Isabella's special care cot so they could be together for the first time. I did this every day for the next month and then Isabella came home. Having them both home at last made it all seem much easier. They were in a good feeding regime set by the hospital and I could then enjoy being mum to twins. 〞

Cath, mum to Alexander and Isabella, eight, born at 27 weeks + four days, weighing 2 lb 3 oz and 2 lb 1 oz respectively; and Oliver, six

Chapter 9

Identical Twins

Being the parent of identical twins gives you unlimited access to a world that doctors, scientists and the general public at large, it sometimes seems, are queuing up to explore.

A twist of genetic fate means that you will spend the rest of your life being asked if your twins have their own language and if they can feel each other's pain. On the plus side, when people ask you if they're identical (as they will – many times), you can answer with a 'yes!', avoiding the unspoken and rather baffling disappointment that 'no' seems to illicit.

Being a parent to identical twins is a fascinating and very special experience, but one in which you can feel alienated, not least because you and your partner may well be the only two people in the world who can reliably tell your children apart. There can be even more doubts and uncertainties about the 'right' way to parent identical twins. How can you help your lovely babies to be confident and independent people while also encouraging their twin bond? What if it all goes wrong and they end up forming a boy band? Worse still: it will all be your fault.

The bad news is that parenting is complicated, fraught with pitfalls, and when things go wrong it will indeed be seen as your fault. The good news is that parenting identical twins is pretty similar to parenting any other child, with just a few tweaks.

Telling your twins apart

When parents-to-be learn they are expecting identical twins, many panic that they won't be able to tell them apart or will muddle them up, causing an identity crisis for life. In fact, the vast majority of parents of identical twins find that they quickly see them as very different babies. Sometimes this is helped by a convenient birthmark or spot, but there can be other clear differences right from the start, such as size or temperament.

However, if your babies are born looking very similar, you may want to try some identifying tactics for the first few weeks or months, such as: keeping on the hospital wristbands, painting the toenails of one twin or having designated clothes for each twin (for example, a special hat or a cardigan – nothing too complicated).

One essential task for new parents of identical twins is to label every photograph. You may think you'll remember that Jonny was wearing the green trousers, but the chances are you won't. In fact, one of the questions that health professionals ask parents of twins who aren't sure whether their children are identical is if they can tell their children apart in photos. Put names to each picture as you take them so that your twins definitely know who they are when they look back at old photos as they grow up.

66 Although by about three months I was confident I could tell the girls apart, my husband wasn't convinced, so sometimes if I'd been out with my son he'd have changed one baby's outfit or done something different just to test if I could still tell who was who. Sometimes it took a few minutes for me to notice, but I usually did! 99

Emma, mum to Amelie and Jessica, 23 months; and Ben, three

66 When they were first born it was really difficult as they were wrapped up with hats on and looked exactly the same. I was really worried about muddling them up and that one of them

would spend their life being the other one! But after about a week at home I felt quite confident and we cut off their hospital tags as they were getting tight anyway. George always has a blue dummy and Archie has a clear dummy – that's how other people tell them apart. I dress them the same every day. They'll probably want to dress differently when they are older, but I just think it's lovely to have them the same. 〞

Alyson, mum to George and Archie, eight months;
and Erin, 12

〝 If the girls are on their own we can't tell who's who and have to put them together. Mia had to have a follow-up blood test and we were halfway through when I realised I'd given them the wrong baby. I almost didn't dare admit it to the doctor, but they found it funny. Now Willow has nail polish on her big toe, just to be sure. 〞

Emily, mum to Willow and Mia, six weeks

How identical will your twins be?

At first glance, identical twins undoubtedly look similar but, although they share the same DNA sequence, they can be surprisingly different, both in personality and physically. In the early days and weeks, it can be difficult to find time to focus on each baby separately, but, when you do, you are likely to start to notice differences in temperament and to see that their responses to the same toys or books can vary dramatically.

The more you are able to focus on each baby individually – and this is not easy, particularly if you have other children to look after, too – the more these individual traits will become apparent, and the more they will help you and others to see them as different people. Try to grab whatever time you can to do this – nappy changing and feeding are good opportunities.

&&Identical twins are born with the same DNA sequence, to the extent that developmental outcomes are genetically influenced. They are more likely to be similar than are other brothers and sisters – including fraternal twins.

However, increasingly we are learning that idiosyncratic differences in the twins' environments and their experiences can contribute to their differences. Because these differences can be very small, they are hard to track systematically – perhaps one twin has colic and cries more than the other when they are very young, and perhaps he or she is picked up more as a consequence, and perhaps this experience very slightly changes their interactions with people and so on. Or perhaps one twin is ill on the first day of nursery and so starts one day later than the other, and perhaps they then have a different key worker who prefers having children do one activity over another. In this way, tiny differences in the environment and how the twins interact with it over time can have an impact on the differences between the children. Just as there are with all children, there are all sorts of experiences that will happen without parents' control. It's true that our environments and experiences can shape who we are, but importantly, we can shape our environments, too. That is, we select, elicit and change our environment and experience throughout our lives. Identical twins are no different.

Parents sometimes fret about what they are or are not doing and how it is affecting their children, and this concern can be exacerbated when you have identical twins as they often become very different people. The important thing to remember is that being an identical twin does not have to be the thing that defines them. Wherever they go, people will be interested in them, and in many respects it might be nice to be seen as so special, but this is not all they are. They are just people, and individuals. To develop to be so, it is important they have some of their own toys, own friends and that they develop individual relationships with parents and siblings, and are not treated as 'the twins' as a unit. 🙶

Dr Bonamy Oliver, developmental psychologist with special expertise in twin families

🙶 They are really close, they don't fight much and seem to enjoy the same things. They still sleep in the same bed. Sometimes we stay somewhere where there are two beds but by the end of the night they've always got into the same one – or mine. Rosa has got a rounder face and Phoenix has got a longer face, but other than that they look exactly the same. Staff at the shoe shop tend to get freaked out because they always have exactly the same shoe size. 🙶

Romany, mum to Rosa and Phoenix, five

🙶 The boys are very similar and very different. The weirdest difference is food. I can understand siblings having different food preferences, but the twins were given exactly the same food at the same times and from the outset Ivor was much fussier and ate a lot less than George. I'd say he probably eats less than half of what George does on a daily basis, but they weigh exactly the same. Our neighbour, who's a GP, uses them as an example to her patients who fuss over their kids' eating habits! 🙶

Lynsey, mum to George and Ivor, six; and Polly, four

Helping others to tell your twins apart

Most parents of identical twins – and eventually the twins themselves – will find that they are frequently asked who's who. Learning to deal with this and coming up with good answers are an essential part of life with identical twins.

You may be surprised by who among your circle of friends and family can tell your twins apart and who finds it difficult. Even close relatives, such as grandparents, can struggle, particularly if they don't see the children regularly, and may feel guilty and slightly embarrassed if they can't work it out. Some people might be good at telling the twins apart when they are together, but not when they see one without the other. It can feel frustrating as a parent to know that the people closest to your children cannot distinguish one from the other. Irritating though it may be, try to throw out some lifelines for those who are struggling to see your children as different people.

Ideas for helping people to identify your identical twins:

▶ Treat your twins as individuals and others are more likely to follow suit.

▶ Don't call them 'the twins'. Gently let anyone who uses that term know that you'd rather they were called by their names.

▶ Try not to always use their names in the same order, to reinforce that they are individuals and that you treat them as such. So say 'Ben and Johnny' just as much as you say 'Johnny and Ben', for fairness.

▶ Use their names frequently so that anyone too embarrassed to ask for a reminder can easily pick up on who's who.

▶ Give grandparents or other close relatives some subtle help if they are struggling. Remind them about differences you know and see; better still, suggest that they look for differences themselves.

▶ Dress the babies in different outfits or, if you prefer to dress them the same, give them different coloured socks or some other small distinguishing detail. When you see or meet people, show them something special about each baby to help reinforce a difference, for example, 'Look at Jacob's lovely new red top' or 'Can you believe how much Millie's hair has grown since you were last here?' This also avoids having to 'officially' say who's who.

66 I don't expect anyone to tell them apart, because I know it's really hard, but I don't like it when people either pretend to know or don't make the effort. When the girls started nursery they were just under one and they each wore a name tag around their wrist. Somebody said I shouldn't name tag them like dogs, but I preferred them to be known by their correct name. We only used them for about a month and then the nursery staff got to know who was who. 99

Emma, mum to Amelie and Jessica, 23 months; and Ben,
three

66 It bothers me that people can't tell them apart in the sense that I don't like it for the girls as I want them to be treated as individuals. I think you have to help people. In school for example, one girl had a centre parting and one had a side parting for their hair. In summer, Aoibheann always has pink sandals and Aileen always yellow (this will continue until they complain). This was also for safety as when they were scooting away from me in the park, I could tell by the shoes which one to call back.

It does have an impact with extra curricular activities that they attend together. They rarely get called by their name and often get overlooked to do something as the demonstrator doesn't know one from the other. We did try sending them at different times but that became a logistical nightmare.

It does bother the girls sometimes. We tend to tell them how special it is to be an identical twin, but this is one of the downsides. Family and close friends know how to tell the girls apart. I think as long as the girls have a sense of themselves as individuals and this is fostered at home and school, the balance is there.

On a funny note, they have told people each other's name on purpose and I think they do enjoy the attention they get. 🙶

Karen, mum to Aileen and Aoibheann, six; and Adam, three

One of the hardest questions for a parent of identical twins to answer is: how do you tell them apart? To the parental eye, the differences are often all too obvious, yet they are also impossible to describe. In the absence of an answer, many people jump in with their own suggestions, which often involve physical comparisons. Someone may judge that one twin has a 'long face' or a 'big head' or a 'small mouth'. While your children are babies, this will have relatively little impact on them, but as they get older it may start to reinforce insecurities about their appearance. Other labels can be equally unhelpful, such as 'Who's the quiet one?' or 'I bet he's the naughty one'. However annoying, coming up with an answer to this persistent question – even if it's a complete lie – will help you stay sane.

Ideas to help you answer the question 'How do you tell them apart?':

▶ 'I find it quite easy, but I appreciate that to most people they look very similar.'

▶ 'It's hard to say, because they change every day. To me, they look very different, but I realise other people find it tricky to see that.'

▶ If you have an older sibling with you, you could try: 'Let's ask the expert. Jamie, how do you tell your sisters apart?'

▶ 'Sometimes it can be hard to tell them apart physically, but they really are very different and that shines through when you know them better.'

Parents tend to assume that older siblings will be able to tell their brothers and sisters apart more easily than adults, and sometimes that is the case. However, quite a few young children are rather baffled by the idea of identical siblings. In the confusion of the first few weeks, some toddlers may not even fully realise that there are two babies, particularly if they are being fed one at a time. Again, give your older child some help by encouraging them to build up a separate relationship with each sibling. This may involve fetching their favourite toy or helping to pick out an outfit. If it can be done safely, encourage your older child to play with one twin nearby while you bath the other twin. They might be able to 'read' them a book, or sing a song to make them laugh. The more siblings get to know the children separately, the more likely they are to see them as different – and therefore not such a force to be reckoned with. Older children may find it upsetting if it is difficult to tell the twins apart for themselves. Reassure him or her that it will get easier as they get older.

66 My son always knows the difference. If you show him a photo, he can always say who is who. One day the girls were looking at a photo of themselves and they were wrong whereas he got it right. 99

Myfanwy, mum to Rojin and Narin, six; and Shivan, nine

66 My daughter Lexi was two when Riley and Henley were born. They were in special care when she came into hospital to meet them. She looked over into Riley's cot and said hello and then climbed up to look at Henley and said: 'No, he's got Riley's eyes – that's Riley.' We had two Rileys for a few weeks after that! 99

Clare, mum to Henley and Riley, 19 months; Lexi, three;
and Kaysie, nine

Chapter 10

Feeding

There cannot be an issue that gives mothers more guilt, pain and anxiety than that of how they feed their babies.

Firstly, let's just be clear: if you are providing your babies with love, milk, lots of cuddles and a regular change of nappy, you are already fulfilling their every need and deserve a massive pat on the back.

Secondly, there are no easy options when it comes to feeding twins. Whether you opt for breast, formula or a bit of both, feeding is a skill that needs to be learnt both by you and your babies. It can be messy, painful, slow, frustrating, confusing and stressful.

Many women who choose to breastfeed their twins are successful, but many more are not. Those who are not can find their dreams and expectations of motherhood crashing down around them as feelings of guilt and failure crowd out a time of bonding and special moments with your new babies.

Women are their own harshest critics, and on this issue never more so. Yet so often they are let down by conflicting advice from health professionals, shunted out of hospital still feeling clueless about how to feed their twins and left to soldier on miserably at home.

Breastfeeding twins is absolutely possible, and can bring you great joy, but to do so successfully requires a huge amount of determination, time and support, which is often sadly lacking from hard-pressed health professionals. Many women begin with huge optimism about breastfeeding, only for their first experience of feeding their twins to turn into a genuinely traumatic sob-fest.

This may not happen to you and if breastfeeding is what you want to do, you will find lots of encouragement and advice in this chapter to help you achieve your goal. If you've decided on formula feeding or switch to this after breastfeeding for a while, you will find just as much encouragement and support. No mother of twins will judge your choices on this issue; convincing yourself to be equally accepting is another matter entirely.

Reality check

Breastfeeding does indeed give your babies the best possible start in life. All that free milk, produced specifically for your babies' needs, is full of nutrients and antibodies to help them fight infection and disease. But that's not the whole picture, particularly where twins are concerned.

Mum after mum reports the mixed messages received from health professionals – being made to feel guilty over inadequate breastfeeding efforts one day and then being pushed to give the babies formula the next. It can be bewildering for women when something that they assumed would be a very natural process proves to be harder than they'd thought, but by that time the hospital doors have long since swung shut and new mums are largely left alone to sort it out themselves.

This is not to advise you to abandon your hopes of breastfeeding – far from it – but on this issue more than any other, being prepared for what lies ahead is key to being successful in feeding your babies the way you choose.

Looking after twins is exhausting, and when you are considering your options, put yourself in the picture, too. Being run ragged and pushed to the edge of your sanity isn't a badge of honour. Sometimes being able to share the feeding load can help you get more rest and therefore enjoy your babies all the more.

Ten points to consider about breastfeeding twins:

1. Allow at least 23 hours a day to feed your newborns. They will probably be on a three-hourly cycle and it may take you two hours to feed them. This will speed up and you will probably learn to feed them together but feeding will be very slow at the start.

2. If you have other children you need to think about how you are going to entertain them during feeding. Breastfeeding while watching your three year old deface the walls rapidly loses its charm. Make contingency entertainment plans with family and friends.

3. Unlike having a single baby, it is not that easy to breastfeed while you are out and about. Unless you enjoy sitting topless in a cafe with a baby hanging off each boob, that is.

4. Breastfeeding is by definition a one-woman job. This can feel like a massive burden or a huge achievement – depending on how much sleep you've had.

5. Research, research, research. Stop any breastfeeding mother of twins and ask them their secrets. Spend hours watching YouTube tandem-feeding videos.

6. It can hurt. No sooner have you got used to having boobs the size and texture of boulders than two small sets of gums are chowing down on them. Cracked nipples and mastitis are excruciating, but by no means inevitable.

7. On a smugness ratio of one to ten, successfully breastfeeding your babies probably comes in at about 200. This may be your greatest achievement.

8 Your breast milk is made exclusively for your babies and gives them all the sustenance they need. It is free, available instantly and at just the right temperature. What's not to like?

9 Your babies have yellow, sweet-smelling poo. Honestly, when you look back, this is good.

10 You and your partner will get very little sleep as you grapple with tiny babies who may not want to latch on or who fall asleep as soon as they do. You will cry, argue and consider divorce. Prepare for this.

Ten points to consider about bottle-feeding twins:

1 You can share feeding with your partner or family.

2 You get more sleep. Sorry, but it's true. Assuming you have someone to share the burden with, you can split feeding into shifts and get four or five hours' kip in a row. Heaven!

3 Guilt. If you can bottle-feed without guilt, you are one in a million.

4 Make space in the kitchen for the military operation that is feeding time. Sterilisers, bottles, teats, extra kettles and tubs of formula will obscure the toaster for some time to come.

5 Feeding two babies formula is not cheap, particularly if you use ready-made cartons when you're out and about.

6 It is easier to get out with your twins, particularly if you use said expensive cartons.

7 You know exactly how much milk your babies have drunk. When they are tiny this is very reassuring.

8 Thousands of babies are bottle-fed every year, and are happy and healthy. You know this, right?

9 Most newborn babies are slow feeders. Allow lots of time for feeding.

10 Bottle-feeding is not an easy option. You will still cry, argue and consider divorcing your partner. Prepare for this.

> ❝I hate how strict the NCT is about breastfeeding, really annoying. On the other hand the NHS sends out a very inconsistent message about what you should be doing and isn't able to provide adequate breastfeeding support. Ultimately you have to work out what you want to do yourself and then find the support you need yourself. You have to be really proactive though about getting what you need because you're on your own!❞
>
> *Helen, mum to Isla and Daisy, four*

> ❝If I'm honest, my heart was never in breastfeeding. My partner and I had talked about it and he fully supported bottle-feeding the girls. We just got on with it.❞
>
> *Alison, mum to Sylvie and Mila, 12 months*

> ❝I let go of a lot of stuff when I knew I was having twins, things about the birth and the pregnancy and there were a lot of little losses. But I still held on to breastfeeding, so when it went so badly it was very hard and very emotional. I still don't think I'm over it.❞
>
> *Alicia, mum to Penny and Abe, six months*

> ❝I breastfed both of them until they were about 13 months old. My incentive for breastfeeding was going to a friend's house when her twins were six weeks old and I was about 34 weeks pregnant, and seeing her husband washing up a million bottles! I hate washing-up. ❞
>
> *Lindsay, mum to Alex and Serafina, 22 months*

Whatever you decide to do, use the experiences of parents in this chapter to help you prepare for the demands of feeding. Allow yourself some wriggle room – you may feel that breastfeeding or bottle-feeding are not for you, but you'll never know until you try it.

Preparing to breastfeed

To breastfeed twins successfully, you need time, confidence, support, cushions and nipples of steel. You also need to be able to withstand many hours of daytime TV or stock up on a lot of box sets. Maximise your chances of managing to breastfeed long term by doing some research well before your babies are due. Knowing what to expect and being prepared to persevere are key to success.

Although breastfeeding is theoretically one of the most natural things in the world, for some it comes more naturally than others. Some babies do just instinctively latch on to the breast in the right position and are away. But for most women there is more work and – be prepared – pain involved before both mummy and babies learn to get it just right. Even women who have breastfed their first or second child find that the transition to twins is not always as straightforward as they'd hoped, although it is great to have the confidence of having already successfully breastfed.

A good starting point is YouTube, which has some brilliant clips of different tandem-feeding techniques posted by twin mums. There are a number of positions you can adopt to feed your twins at the same time.

Tandem breastfeeding positions include:

▸ **Football or rugby hold** – In this position you essentially have a baby under each arm. It is a good one to start with as the babies' feet are out of the way and you can concentrate on getting a good latch.

▸ **Cradle hold** – The classic breastfeeding position if you were to have one baby. With two, you can feed one from each side and cradle them together with legs and bodies overlapping in front of you. This can mean having to support the babies with your arms, which is tiring, and when they get a bit bigger they are likely to kick each other, so it is best used when they are very small.

▸ **A bit of both** – Have one baby in the football or rugby hold to one side of you and the other in the cradle hold.

▸ **Reclining** – Prop yourself up on pillows and adopt any of the holds above. Some women find this more comfortable than sitting up and more manageable than lying down.

▸ **Lying down** – Try lying on your side with a pillow behind your back and bum. One baby can lie on its side on the bed against you and the other can lie across your body with its feet towards its sibling.

Breastfeeding mums differ over which cushion formation works for them. Some prefer the pyramid approach: piling ordinary cushions around them and nestling the babies on top. Other mums could not be without a specific twins breastfeeding pillow – designs vary but they are moulded into a horseshoe shape that fits around you and then does up with a clip. Rather like an armchair, this has the advantage of holding the babies at a perfect height for most boobs and allows you to feed them, one from each side, hands free. When you are more experienced, you can feed one while burping the other. Or, even better, feed both while operating the remote control and shovelling cake into your mouth.

Until your babies are born, you won't know what will work for you, so it's probably advisable not to race out and buy a lot of expensive and bulky equipment. You can often pick up twin feeding pillows second hand.

Accept that feeding your babies will take time. Initially you are likely to be feeding every three hours. As it can take more than an hour to feed and wind each baby, you could be spending two out of every three hours sitting and feeding. You may learn to feed them together and the babies themselves will feed faster, so it does speed up.

The most important thing to remember is that breastfeeding is not supposed to hurt. If you experience pain when you latch on then use your finger to release your baby's suction and start again. A bad latch will lead to sore and cracked nipples. If you are unlucky you may experience blocked milk ducts or mastitis, which are quite possibly the most painful things you will ever endure. And this is written in the full knowledge that you've just given birth. However, it doesn't happen to everybody and the more research you do in advance and the more support you have, the less likely it is to strike. (See later in this chapter for advice on how to deal with common breastfeeding problems.)

It is important to have an effective support network. Firstly, make sure you and your partner agree about feeding and are aware that the early days will be difficult. Being exhausted, uncertain and anxious is not an ideal starting line for an early-hours discussion about why one or both of the twins won't latch on, so be prepared for tears and accusations to be shed and uttered in conditions of extreme duress. This is a really hard time for everyone, especially partners who have to stand on the sidelines watching the person they love in pain and struggling with feelings of failure if all does not go to plan. Finding the right thing to say can feel impossible.

There is lots of help available in the community, both free and paid for. Search in your area for independent breastfeeding counsellors or breastfeeding support groups. As with anything else, you will identify with some and back away from others. Give yourself time to talk to people before the babies come so you have a clear idea of who will be of most help to you, should you need it. Go with your instincts: do you like and trust this person? Do they make you feel comfortable? Visit your nearest twins group for more first-hand advice on feeding. These mums may also have good recommendations for local support networks. Your local hospital may run antenatal classes for multiples, which will cover feeding, but this very much depends on where you live.

> **❝** I was determined to breastfeed and had read up a lot about it. I had also contacted a few volunteer breastfeeding counsellors in advance of the girls' birth, so that I knew who to ring if anything went wrong and when it did they were fantastic. **❞**
>
> *Helen, mum to Isla and Daisy, four*

Breastfeeding your twins is a very special gift to them. It is a wonderful way to bond with your babies and allows you to rest as you sit or lie with them feeding either individually or together. Breastfeeding also lowers your risk of getting breast and ovarian cancer, and apparently burns up in excess of 500 calories a day – although this may be offset by the amount of food you eat in return.

Feeding in hospital

So much energy is expended speculating about the likely pain levels in giving birth to two babies that it can come as something of a shock to find that your babies have arrived and there's still more work to do.

In an ideal world, your babies should be suckling within an hour of birth. At this stage you are not producing milk but colostrum, a thick, sticky and yellowish liquid high in carbohydrates, protein and antibodies. If you have to express colostrum to give it to your babies in the neonatal unit, don't be disappointed to find you have only produced what appears to be a minute thimbleful. Colostrum provides its nutrients in a very concentrated form, so every drop really does count.

In this slightly dazed, spaced-out and joyful period, you will probably still be reliving the birth and persuading your brain to catch up with the fact that the big bump has now become two babies. Hopefully your babies are with you but it may be that one or both twins have had to be taken to the special care unit, in which case there is an air of unreality and obvious concern. (See the next section for feeding premature babies in hospital.)

If you have one or both of the babies with you, your midwife should be helping you latch the babies on. Don't be surprised if it's not as easy as you thought, even if you have spent hours studying ideal latch positions. This is normal. You are not useless – you are a new mother of twins who hasn't done this before. Get help and ask for more if you don't think it feels right. It is really important to get a correct latch straight away to try to minimise sore nipples.

Tips to get a good latch:

- Hold your baby close with its nose to your nipple

- Wait until your baby opens its mouth really wide – you can encourage this by stroking their top lip

- Bring your baby on to your breast. The baby should have a large mouthful of breast and you shouldn't see much (if any) nipple

- You should see and feel a rhythmic sucking. Your baby's lower jaw will be working up and down as it sucks

Get your partner to go and look for help if none is offered. At this stage there are trained staff around and it is easier to get people's attention, so take advantage of it. In the early hours and days, offer the babies your breast as and when they want it.

66 When the babies were born, nearly four weeks early and by C-section, they were both breastfed by me in the recovery room, mostly thanks to my midwives propping them up with pillows and tucking their bodies, rugby ball like, under my arms. 99

Amanda, mum to Freya and Casper, two; Gabriel, seven; and Felix, ten

66 I had been told by almost every midwife I had met that breastfeeding twins immediately after an epidural was practically impossible. It isn't. I had enough sensation in my legs after twenty minutes to sit up and breastfeed both girls. They were kind enough to demand feeding one by one! 99

Helen, mum to Sophia and Hannah, three

> 66 I started to shake quite violently which is apparently a common reaction to an epidural, but I hadn't been warned about it. My teeth were chattering and I was really juddering. At the same time a student nurse was trying to get me to breastfeed. She had never done it before and wasn't even getting paid for the day. She stood over me with the babies, trying to get them to latch on, but she didn't know what she was doing. It was traumatic and I had to almost shout at her that I wasn't well enough to do this before she would stop. 99
>
> *Alison, mum to Sylvie and Mila, 12 months*

Meanwhile, those of you whose twins are already feeding (or sometimes even if they are not) will be heading out of the recovery room and down to the postnatal ward. As we have already discussed in Chapter 7, the postnatal ward is generally not the friend of a twin mum, with staff stretched to the limit, and sometimes lacking expertise and understanding of the specific needs of twin parents. Hopefully your local hospital will be the honourable exception to this rule, but the chances are it won't. So, shout, cry and beg for a private room and do the same to ensure your partner is allowed to stay. Many couples decide that their partner will go home to get some rest for the first night, assuming that mum will have the support she needs in hospital. Others are turfed out, regardless of what they want to do. This can leave a new mum, possibly almost immobile after a C-section, with next to no support for her first night attempting to breastfeed her twins.

If staff are worried about your babies not putting on enough weight, it will sometimes be suggested that you feed them formula using a small cup. You sit up one baby at a time and give them tiny sips from this cup.

 When I was in hospital on the first night, there was no breastfeeding support and the night staff didn't have time to help me, they tried to push me to bottle-feed. I saw a breastfeeding counsellor the following morning by which time I was in a terrible state, and she got me back on track in terms of showing me what to do but in the end I did start feeding them formula using a cup as well as breastfeeding because of the pressure that the care staff were putting on me – telling me that I didn't have enough milk and doubting whether it was possible to breastfeed both of them. Initially they wouldn't let my partner stay in the hospital, but I argued that as they didn't have the resources to help me, it was only fair that they let him stay. Eventually they let him sleep on a roll mat and they gave us a room, which was much better than being on the ward.

Helen, mum to Isla and Daisy, four

 I was left unattended and unchecked on my own in a private room from 9 p.m. till 6 a.m. Hannah had fed well overnight, but Sophia had slept through almost completely. No one had actually told me what I ought to be doing or that I should be waking the babies to feed every three hours, and the midwife who saw me at 6 a.m. basically freaked out. She did a blood test on Sophia and it showed she had low blood sugar. I just didn't have enough milk or anything at this point to reverse the situation. I was told that low blood sugar could affect brain development, so the only solution was to introduce other milk – in this case, breast milk usually reserved for special care baby unit (SCBU) babies. So I started combining my own breastfeeding with other women's breast milk, not through a bottle but cup feeding. We had to clasp these tiny babies under the neck and tilt a minute cup towards their lips in the hope they would automatically swallow. This combined cup and breastfeeding continued for the entire seven days

I was in hospital and yet still their blood sugar seemed all over the place. Eventually it levelled and we went home – where our community midwife told us to stop using cups and move on to bottles. By this time the girls had been moved on to formula, which I think hugely hampered my attempts to breastfeed. 〝

Helen, mum to Hannah and Sophia, three

〝 I had mixed help in hospital, but mainly encouragement. Since I'd breastfed before and had gone to a few refresher classes whilst pregnant, I was fairly confident. Some midwives were great and others not. In hospital I often had to get in and out of bed with both my babies on my own (despite having had a C-section); there was not much assistance on hand and you had to wait so long for a response from the ward team that it was necessary to just get on with it. I managed to prop the babies in my arms safely in bed so I could sleep sitting up and feed them on demand and at least every three hours. 〝

Jackie, mum to Tristan and Sebastian, three; and Isla, ten

Feeding premature babies

Having newborn twins in a hospital special care unit can be both terrifying and reassuring. Knowing that your tiny babies are in the best possible hands is immensely comforting, yet seeing them in an alien, beeping unit can make parents feel helpless.

Feeding can help mothers reassert some element of control over their babies' care. Providing your twins with expressed colostrum and, later, milk, is something that only you can do and it gives them unique nutrients that really benefit their development. For mothers who have one or both of their babies in the hospital's special care unit, expressing colostrum becomes the order of the day (and night). To some, using a breast pump can feel uncomfortably close to milking time, and doing so in the proximity of other women in the hospital's expressing room can be intimidating, although others enjoy the camaraderie. It is necessary to pump very regularly, every two to two and a half hours around the clock, to ensure that your milk flow is established.

66 When the girls were first born and were in NICU (the neonatal intensive care unit), I was very keen to express colostrum for them. The first few days were a real struggle, and I found it difficult to express anything much. I was in the routine of trying every two to three hours so, on my second night in hospital I dutifully woke at 3 a.m. After much squeezing and sobbing, I finally managed to fill a pitifully small vial. In my complete daze of half consciousness, putting the lid on became the next hurdle. I somehow managed to catch the vial with my arm and knocked the entire contents over the table. I was absolutely devastated. 99

Maeve, mum to Maia and Iona, five, born at 31 weeks

66 The nurses were on at me all the time about expressing. You're in a tiny room with other women oozing like cows. I wanted to tell the nurses to just lay off – I was doing the best I could. 99

Neela, mum to Mohan and Rohan, 23 months, born at 34 weeks; and Asha, four

66 I had talked about feeding to the hospital before the babies were born. I didn't want to breastfeed them but the hospital was adamant that this was what they had to have if they

were born prem. They said breast milk was like 'golden nectar' for the babies. I agreed they could use donor breast milk and then thought I'd try to express but my milk never came through. After three weeks of donor milk they were weaned on to formula. 〞

Anna, mum to Mia and Sam, seven months, born at 30 weeks; Harry, ten; and Olivia, 13

Depending on the prematurity and health of your babies, they may be fed using an intravenous line (which goes directly into a vein) or through either a nasal or mouth tube. Even if your babies can digest milk, they are unlikely to be mature enough to coordinate swallowing, sucking and breathing until about 32 to 34 weeks. Babies can suck from about 28 weeks and will be encouraged to do so, using a dummy or the tip of your finger, to prepare for feeding through their mouths.

It is not uncommon to be able to express well for your babies but to find it hard to make the transition from the babies taking breast milk from a bottle to taking milk directly from the breast. This can require a lot of perseverance.

One of the few bonuses about having your babies in special care is that you leave hospital with an established, regular feeding routine, which is a comforting thing to cling on to when faced with the uncertainty of caring for your two fragile-seeming new arrivals. No matter how good your babies' care is, as their health and strength improves, you will be anxious that they hit their weight and feeding targets so you can get them home. That in itself can add to your stress, particularly if you have had one baby discharged already.

> 66 You are just desperate for them to put on weight so you can get them out of hospital. They were weighed each week, which became a focal point. 99
>
> *Jennifer, mum to Isabella and Alexander, five months, born at 31 weeks + four days*

You will probably find that your babies are still having formula feeds to top up your breastfeeding, using either cups or bottles, when they are discharged from hospital, but this doesn't mean that it is not possible to exclusively breastfeed once they have become a little stronger.

> 66 You will be able to exclusively breastfeed gradually at home. As they get stronger feeders you will be able to drop to three top-ups a day and then once you've 'proved' they're putting on weight you can drop all of them. It's a gradual process. A lot of mums manage to drop all the top-ups a couple of weeks down the line. 99
>
> *Kathryn, mum to Drew and Jevan, nine; Kier, four; and Marty five weeks. Kathryn is also an ABM (Association of Breastfeeding Mothers) breastfeeding counsellor*

Feeding at home

The first few weeks of feeding your babies at home are undoubtedly some of the most stressful times you will experience. You will be grappling with the logistics of how to feed two babies, managing painful and huge boobs, and worrying about whether your twins are putting on weight, all while suffering from extreme fatigue.

Try not to panic. Babies lose weight after birth and can take two weeks, sometimes more, to regain their birth weight. Feeding your babies takes some getting used to and no one gets it right straight away. Remember that feeding will become quicker and easier. Your milk operates on a supply-and-demand basis, so the more sucking and demand your boobs receive, the more milk they will supply. Feed often to firmly establish the milk supply.

We will look at general tips on how to manage at home in Chapter 11, but here are a few pointers for feeding in the early days.

Ten tips for feeding in the first few days at home:

1. Make sure your partner knows as much about breastfeeding and/or bottle-feeding as you do. It is too much to expect one person to make all the decisions.

2. Agree with your partner before the babies arrive how you want to feed them and discuss how you will do this as a team. If breastfeeding, your partner can change each baby, bring them to you and help you latch on, then wind the babies after feeding. If bottle-feeding, one person can prepare the bottles and you can feed and wind one twin each.

3. Have the confidence to stick to your plan for a while. Friends, relatives and medical staff will have their opinions, but give your plan a go – it might just work.

4. Initially, feeding will take up most of your day. This cannot be overemphasised.

5. Try to make sure that someone other than your partner is there to look after you all. Your partner will probably be up all night with you – you will both need help.

6. There will be times in the middle of the night when both babies are crying and you can't work out why. They will have been fed, burped and changed, but still they are howling. It is at this point of exhaustion that you will question whether you can carry on, continue to be married to your partner or ever be a successful parent. You can, honestly. Just get through one night at a time.

7. Grab any opportunity to sleep.

8. Experiment with feeding positions. Some will work for you and others won't. When you find the right position feeding will seem a lot easier.

9. Keep everything you will need during feeding within reach as you will be immobile for a while. Always have a muslin cloth handy – feeding can be messy.

10. Bottle-fed babies are perfectly happy and healthy. Let go of the guilt and do what works for your family.

At this stage, do not stress about getting your babies into any sort of routine – it is too early. Concentrate on breastfeeding often.

Eating well and drinking lots of water will help your milk supply. There are certain foods (called 'lactogenic') that are known to boost milk supply, such as oats, spinach, carrots, papaya, asparagus and dried apricots. It is also thought that almonds, and seeds such as sesame, pumpkin and sunflower, can help your supply. Keep an eye on your diet for another reason, too – mothers report that their consumption of onions, cauliflower, broccoli, beans and garlic can cause extra wind in their babies.

66 The best advice I have is to persevere with tandem feeding. It's a pain, and you feel like a sow with piglets, but it is worth it. Otherwise it's all you ever do. The other thing, though, is to embrace mixed feeding – mine were bottle refusers and it would have been lovely to have been able to give formula occasionally. 99

Lindsay, mum to Alex and Serafina, 22 months

66 I beat myself up about formula, but I could see that my babies had to eat and drink and I realised that it didn't matter. You have to appreciate your babies and if you worry too much about breastfeeding that moment will pass. 99

Pornthida, mum to Art and Enda, five months

66 I was trying to breastfeed Jed, then bottle-feed him, then offer Millie the breast and afterwards bottle-feed her and then express with the pump for later. It meant the session was taking three hours. I couldn't work out why I was so tired and desperate and tearful. It just wasn't doable. When I realised I wasn't going to breastfeed there was a sense of relief – as well as sadness and guilt. Feeding became less stressful; we could feed both babies in an hour and a quarter, and could enjoy it rather than it feeling like an endless traumatic round. We felt that maybe this could work. 99

Mercedes, mum to Millie and Jed, two weeks

66 I had to keep notes when I was feeding them, as to when, for how long, which breast and so on, since they were not always awake at the same time for double feeding. When they were asleep, I would express and build up stocks in the freezer, just in case I got ill or needed help with feeding. This had the additional effect of keeping my milk production

going. Breastfeeding two hungry babies exclusively had the advantage of increasing my milk production. I only stopped breastfeeding them when they started fighting over my breasts whilst holding on to both my nipples with their teeth! 🙼

Jackie, mum to Tristan and Sebastian, three; and Isla, ten

🙼 Trying to get a baby to take nourishment and comfort six times a day when it has been used to being fed constantly in the womb is quite a lot to expect. Babies can't read clocks. They're hungry when they're hungry. 🙼

Kathryn, mum to Drew and Jevan, nine; Kier, four; and Marty five weeks. Kathryn is also an ABM (Association of Breastfeeding Mothers) breastfeeding counsellor

Bottle-feeding at home

Formula milk is not sterile, and this has prompted a series of increasingly stringent guidelines about how to prepare bottles with the least risk of bacterial contamination. The latest recommendations are to prepare bottles on demand, with water that has only just been boiled, and to cool the bottles quickly before giving them to your babies. It is not recommended to heat bottles in the microwave as this may create hotspots that could burn your babies' mouths.

It is probably fair to say that anyone who has experienced the double howl of newborns – or any other stage for that matter – will be frowning as they read this advice. Or possibly howling, too. Waiting for the kettle to boil at 3 a.m., making up the bottles and then attempting to cool the bottles again, all against the backdrop of two hungry babies wanting their milk, is almost certainly something that Department of Health officials will never have experienced.

The new guidelines may not seem new-twin-parent friendly but they are based on real health concerns which should not be ignored.

The World Health Organization's bottle-feeding recommendations:

► Use boiled water originally taken from the cold tap

► Pour the boiled water (no cooler than 70°C, so it should not have been left in the kettle for more than 30 minutes) into a cleaned and sterilised bottle

► Add the exact amount of formula to the water in the bottle

► Mix thoroughly by gently shaking and swirling the bottle

► Immediately cool to feeding temperature by holding the bottle under cold running water or by placing in a container of cold or iced water

► Check the temperature by dripping a little on to the inside of your wrist. It should feel lukewarm, not hot

► Throw away any feed that has not been consumed within two hours

The WHO issued the following advice about bottles that need to be made up in advance, which may be of some comfort:

"It is safest to prepare a fresh feed each time one is needed, and to consume immediately. This is because prepared feeds provide ideal conditions for bacteria to grow – especially when kept at room temperature. If you need to prepare feeds in advance for use later, they should be prepared in individual bottles, cooled quickly and placed in the refrigerator (no higher than 5°C).'

Throw away any refrigerated feed that has not been used within 24 hours. "

WHO's Food Safety Guidance,
How to Prepare Formula for Bottle-feeding at Home

All parents who bottle-feed stress the need to be well organised. Most have a separate kettle just for making up feeds and all have a system for washing, sterilising and storing bottles and teats to ensure clean and sterile apparatus is always to hand.

"I bought 16 bottles because I didn't know what I was doing, but I probably use eight. I make up two to three feeds in advance and keep them in the fridge.

I sit on a futon which slopes at a slight angle and have one baby on each side by my legs. Alexander feeds really well so I can sometimes roll up a muslin and prop up the bottle so I've got a free hand to have a cup of tea or use the remote control. "

Jennifer, mum to Isabella and Alexander, five months

"Bottle-feeding is one of those things you have to be organised about – get it all ready in advance and then the babies scream for less time. It was a well-oiled machine within a few weeks. "

Helen, mum to Hannah and Sophia, three

> 66 Initially we did eight feeds a day, but 16 bottles take up a lot of space so we made do with eight. We had a microwave steriliser and a bottle drainer that just stood on the draining board that was really useful. I learnt who was more patient and would start with the other one, or give a bit of milk and then give them their dummy and give the other one some of their bottle. When they were old enough to sit in the bouncy chairs I'd sit on the floor between them and feed them together like that. 99
>
> *Alison, mum to Sylvie and Mila, 12 months*

Formula-fed babies

So many parents have so much to say about bottle-feeding, and yet compiling this section was arguably the most difficult part of the book. Many tips and suggestions now contravene current guidelines, although at the time were adopted in good faith and often at the suggestion of health professionals. The current advice on preparing bottles is based on genuine health concerns arising from the fact that formula milk is not sterile and this should be respected. To clarify this further, have a more detailed discussion with your health visitor about ways in which to ensure you can always and safely have a bottle ready for your hungry babies.

Mixed feeding

So polarised is the debate about breastfeeding versus bottle-feeding that it is slightly surprising to find that it isn't a black and white issue at all. For many parents of twins, mixed feeding provides the perfect balance between exclusive breastfeeding and exclusive bottle-feeding. Mixed feeding allows you to carry on giving your babies breast milk but spreads the load a little by building in some formula feeds.

Mothers are often put off mixed feeding because health professionals warn of 'nipple confusion', where once babies have been shown a bottle they will reject the breast. This can happen, but there are many, many stories of successful mixed feeding and, if you feel ready to abandon breastfeeding through sheer exhaustion or are simply looking for a new approach, this is an option worth considering.

66 A lot of mums find success with alternating breastfeeds and formula feeds. Some mums prefer to breastfeed at night and do more formula in the day. Some mums prefer to formula feed when out and about. Some mums prefer to breastfeed when out and about so they don't need to remember to take all the bottle-feeding gubbins. Whatever you decide, as long as you do roughly the same thing every day your milk supply will adjust. Remember it's demand and supply so whatever your babies demand your breasts will provide, whether that be fully breastfeeding, breastfeeding four feeds a day or doing two a day. It's completely up to you. 99

Kathryn, mum to Drew and Jevan, nine; Keir, four; and Marty, five weeks. Kathryn is also an ABM (Association of Breastfeeding Mothers) breastfeeding counsellor

66 I exclusively breastfed them for six weeks, by which time I was exhausted and we introduced a night-time bottle of formula, followed by another, given to them by my husband, so that I could get some sleep. This worked really well and we continued with this until they were about three or four months and only waking once in the night, and then I took over but continued with

the formula at night-time. I carried on breastfeeding during the day until they were about nine months. 〞

Amanda, mum to Freya and Casper, three; Gabriel, seven; and Felix, ten

〝 You need so much milk to feed two babies – I felt I wasn't designed for it. It was taking so much time and was so restrictive. I just felt it wasn't fair on the rest of my family, so at five weeks we introduced one to two bottles a day, which worked well. 〞

Elsa, mum to Lulu and Abigail, four months; Luke, two; and Tom, four

Troubleshooting feeding issues

It seems that no sooner have you got yourself into a feeding pattern than a new hurdle approaches. Don't despair. All the conditions mentioned here are common and, although often hell at the time, do pass and are treatable. Many twin mums report that their GPs were not very well attuned to these problems, so go to your surgery prepared with some research of your own or be persistent if you feel that things aren't right. Remember that you know yourself and your babies better than anyone else.

Cracked or bleeding nipples

Getting a good latch is vital to avoid painful and bleeding nipples. If there is pain when your babies latch on, then release their grip by putting your finger into their mouths and start again. They should have a good mouthful of boob, including most or all of the nipple, and you will see their jaws working as they drink the milk.

Tips for avoiding and dealing with cracked nipples:

▶ Squeeze a few drops of breast milk, which is believed to have minor healing properties, on to your nipples at the end of your feed

▶ Let your nipples dry after each feed

▶ Wear a cotton bra so air can circulate

▶ Change breast pads at each feed. Preferably don't use breast pads with a plastic backing

▶ Treat cracks with soft paraffin or purified lanolin. Put ointment on the crack only

Mastitis

Mastitis occurs when breast tissue becomes inflamed, producing pain in your boobs which ranges from excruciating to absolutely unbearable. It is caused by an infection or milk remaining in the milk tissue. You may also feel a lump, called a blocked duct, which is the build-up of milk in your breast. As well as extreme pain and swollen boobs, you will have flu-like feelings, such as a high temperature, aches and chills.

All your instincts tell you to protect your breast from gnawing babies, but it's really important to keep feeding despite the agony, because more milk left in the breast will make matters worse. Antibiotics can be prescribed if symptoms persist.

Tips for avoiding and dealing with mastitis:

▶ Gently stroke the breast towards the nipple while feeding

▶ Comb breast with wide-tooth comb (this gets into the ducts)

▶ Use a cold compress to ease the swelling

▶ Place warm flannels on the breast before feeding to get the milk flowing

▶ Expressing from the affected breast can be easier to bear

▶ Express in the bath or shower

▶ Take ibuprofen for pain, temperature and inflammation

❝I had really painful blocked ducts and a blocked nipple pore. I felt pain in my breast and then when I was feeding I actually felt the lump move to my nipple. It was like a blob of congealed milk blocking the nipple. In the end it went away after a few weeks through feeding – like an iceberg dissolving. ❞

Lucy, mum to Jack and Iona, five months; Sam, three; and Beth, five

❝I did notice that, feeding two, my body would often go a bit mad on the production. Several times at night I woke up leaking, engorged, fevery and shaky [the precursor to mastitis] but a scalding hot shower in the middle of the night, some Nurofen and drinking plenty of water kept it at bay. ❞

Tracy, mum to Toren and Mairead, six; Edan, two; and Conall, ten

---

Thrush

The warm moistness of your babies' mouths combined with the sugar in milk means that feeding mothers often get thrush on their nipples or breasts, which is extremely painful. In turn, babies get thrush in their mouths. This is a fungal infection and must be treated by a doctor because otherwise you and your babies will continue to pass it to each other.

Tips for avoiding and dealing with thrush:

▶ Cut down your sugar intake

▶ Wash clothes and bedding at 60°C

▶ Sterilise everything a baby sucks – even toys

▶ Consider taking acidophilus capsules, which restore bacteria that naturally keep thrush at bay

> My GP was absolutely useless, at one point when I had thrush on one breast I was advised to feed both babies on the other breast! He had no idea. I think the biggest lesson for me was that you have to manage your own care and find any information yourself, then communicate what you want to medical professionals in no uncertain terms!
>
> *Helen, mum to Isla and Daisy, three*

Tongue tie

Tongue tie happens when the skin that attaches the tongue to the base of the mouth is unusually short and tight, restricting the tongue's movement. This affects 3–10 per cent of newborns and can mean they have serious problems latching on. It should be identified by your health visitor or GP and can be easily dealt with while babies are very young.

Reflux

Reflux is a very common problem but one that causes parents immense anguish. There is nothing more disheartening than having got milk down your baby only to see it thrown up and to have an unhappy, grizzling child on your hands. Seeing your baby (or maybe babies) in pain and feeling that you can't do anything about it is very hard to deal with. Reflux is all about immaturity in the muscles around the baby's food pipe, which connects the mouth with the stomach. Reflux occurs when the valve that lets through the swallowed milk hasn't developed sufficiently and allows milk and stomach acid to come back up, causing discomfort.

The problem with reflux is that it is a bit of a catch-all condition, with many different treatments, so it requires perseverance with your GP if the first medication doesn't seem to be effective. It can also mask other issues, such as allergies. Some parents find that their babies did not have reflux as originally diagnosed, but a type of milk intolerance, such as an allergy to milk protein. Remember that it is not normal for babies to be in pain and crying for the majority of the day. If this is happening, seek medical help and don't be fobbed off.

Tips for avoiding and dealing with reflux:

► Keep the baby upright during and after feeds

► Use slings or bouncy chairs to keep the babies upright during the day

► Raise the cot or Moses basket at the head end to help at night or during naps

> ❝Reflux was horrific. I had no idea what was wrong, I just thought Alex was colicky, or a 'shouty baby' in the words of my health visitor. Then when he was about three months old one of my friends was round and watched him feeding – with the screaming, arching, vomiting that entailed – and suggested I take him to the GP. We were given Gaviscon, which was impossible to deliver, then ranitidine. After about two days he suddenly switched into a normal baby, and I've only heard that awful scream of pain since when he trapped his finger in a drawer. He started sleeping properly, feeding normally, and was just a much happier little soul. I feel awful that it took us so long to get him sorted out, but am so grateful we did.❞
>
> *Lindsay, mum to Alex and Serafina, 22 months*

Constipation

This is rarely a problem with breastfed babies, but is quite common if your babies are being formula fed. The easiest way to deal with this is by giving the babies a small amount of cooled, boiled water before each feed (30–40 ml). If this doesn't work, see your health visitor.

> ❝After we got them home they got quite constipated. When I mentioned this to our health visitor a few days later she told me they should have water by itself to deal with it. No one had told us and we felt really upset and like bad parents just because we didn't know. Water really helped and made getting their wind up easier, too. Now we give them two ounces before every feed.❞
>
> *Emily, mum to Willow and Mia, six weeks*

Wind

Winding twins tends to be an afterthought, a small sign-off to lengthy feeding rituals. What no one warns you about is that if you duly hoist your baby on to your shoulder and pat its back, a big fat burp does not always follow automatically. In fact, you can sometimes spend as long trying to wind your baby as you have feeding it. When you are tired and you've got another baby to go, this can often be the last straw.

Be aware that if you eat certain foods – such as garlic, onions, beans, broccoli and cauliflower – it can cause extra wind in your babies.

Without winding, your babies are likely to be awake again soon with uncomfortable tummies, so don't be tempted to take shortcuts. Try lots of different positions for winding and hopefully you'll find one that works.

Alternative positions for speedy winding:

1. Lay your baby along one arm (head at elbow, legs dangling either side of your arm) and pat its back. You can sit or walk round like this (making sure the baby doesn't fall off, obviously).

2. Put your baby on your shoulder and go up and down the stairs.

3. Lay your baby on its back and cycle its legs.

4. Lay your baby on its front on your leg and rub its back. You can use this position for tandem burping – sit on the floor with legs outstretched and lay both babies across them on their tummies, rubbing their backs.

5. Sit your baby upright on your knee, putting your hand on its chest and gently supporting its throat, then pat or rub its back.

6 You can also bounce your baby gently on your knee or try gently rotating the baby's upper body in this upright, sitting position.

7 Lay your baby down on a hard surface (such as a table or the floor rather than a bed), sit it up again and try to burp using your favourite position.

Chapter 11

Home Alone

Leaving hospital and embarking on your next giant step for familykind is a thrilling moment. Finally it is just you and your babies – life as you've never known it starts here. In the hospital car park, to be precise, as you placate two tiny babies whose first memories may well be of you swearing at their car seats.

Don't be surprised to find that it is well past your bedtime (i.e. 7 p.m.), because despite keeping your babies in suffocating temperatures in the wards, hospitals think nothing of discharging you and your little ones late into the night, often after making you hang around for hours while an elusive consultant is tracked down to sign you off.

However late, early, protracted or scarily quick your hospital discharge proves to be, you have cleared a massive hurdle. You've gained your freedom, piled on a bit more responsibility and have taken a step towards parental independence.

> 66 I felt a huge sense of relief that I was not in the noisy hospital ward any longer. It was great being in a familiar environment and to get to know Tommy and Lizzie. I felt much more in control and a lot less stressed and breastfeeding started to come more easily. 99
>
> *Linda, mum to Tommy and Lizzie, 11 months*

"It was terrifying leaving hospital. I thought we'd be all excited, but I would have been happy to stay there forever. We were discharged after four days, which was just at the point when hormones spike, so I was super weepy anyway. We'd bought them some little hoodies and I kept crying and saying they looked like they were ready to go to university. My mom kept reminding me that they were 5 lb. She clearly thought I was ridiculous. "

Alicia, mum to Penny and Abe, six months

"We had our own room in hospital which was great but became a bit like a prison. When we were released after five days I felt like that bloke from *The Shawshank Redemption* – I had this sense of liberation and kept looking up at the sky and breathing in fresh air! "

Ming, dad to Alfred and Joseph, two

If one or both of your babies has been in special care for a while, you may have got into a regular feeding pattern but, for the majority of babies, routine is something that may come quite a bit later.

For now, it is about managing each day at a time and establishing a way of doing things that suits your family. As discussed in Chapter 10, you will be feeding on demand, and much of the first few weeks will be spent feeding, winding and changing nappies. It is a slow process to start with. Prepare for the fact that being in hospital in no way constitutes a rest, so you will be exhausted, as will your partner, who, with luck, will have been able to support you on the ward. You may well have other children to share your focus and who do not understand how much time the new babies will demand of Mummy and Daddy.

Having extra pairs of hands at home at this stage is essential. You all need to be looked after and you need time to find ways of making feeding work and establishing how best to settle the babies.

Tips to prepare you for the first night at home with twins:

► Accept that you are unlikely to get any sleep. The babies will either cry all night or they will sleep – either way you will be so anxious you'll be awake.

► At least as you lie awake you can listen to your own children rather than the nurses' plans for the weekend.

► Your partner won't know why they're crying either.

► If you make it to 24 hours home alone without a monumental, teary meltdown, it's an amazing achievement!

► Finding a feeding position that works at night takes time. Don't despair if you don't arrive at it straight away. Keep experimenting with feeding and burping positions. Remember: this is the slowest that the changing/feeding/winding process will ever be.

► You will cope and you can do it. Honestly, you can.

‟ We got back at 7 p.m. and it was dark and freezing cold because we hadn't been home for a week. We had no food – not even bread and milk. We were obsessed by the girls either freezing or overheating, and had thermometers in every room. We had all this stuff and yet none of it seemed to be what we needed. In the end we phoned a friend who had triplets and she basically completely rearranged our house, moved the cots and told us what to do. It was brilliant! 〝

Gabby, mum to Astrid and Florrie, 12 weeks

〝 When we got back, they just would not stop crying. I'd not established good feeding with either of them, but we didn't know whether they were hungry, or tired, or what. We put them down, they cried, we picked them up, they cried. We ended up sitting up in bed, with all the lights on, me trying endlessly to get them to latch on, crying my eyes out, snot streaming down my face, and just thinking 'What have we done?' We eventually got to sleep and a little while later my husband woke up freaking out, hunting under the duvet trying to find one of them. We checked, and they were both fast asleep in their cot. We were completely delirious and one of us had put them down without even remembering. The first few nights followed a very similar pattern, but we got there eventually. 〝

Lynsey, mum to Ivor and George, four; and Polly 18 months

〝 When we brought them home, I remember the feeling of my babies finally being mine. Before that point it had felt as though I wasn't truly their mother, because nurses and doctors and other people were doing the majority of care. I also remember feeling very scared and unsure of what I was doing. I was overwhelmingly happy though – and spent most of the night just staring at them sleeping. 〝

Natalie, mum to Gabriel and Cerys, two

Attempting to determine why your children are crying and then doing something to make it stop will take up a fair chunk of your time for the foreseeable future, but never more so than at this early stage, when you understandably lack the confidence to interpret their tears and assume, sometimes correctly, that something must be wrong. Hunger, wind, uncomfortable nappies and tiredness are the obvious first ports of call. If you suspect illness because of a temperature or rash or worrying signs of any sort, you must seek urgent medical help. Often, though, your babies are simply unsettled and you may never work out why.

Ideas for settling your babies:

▸ **Swaddling** – A technique of snugly wrapping up your babies which simulates the cosiness of the womb and which many babies find comforting. Make sure your cotton sheet wraps them snugly but not so firmly that it restricts all movement, as a recent study has shown links between swaddling and developmental hip dysplasia. Studies also suggest a possible increased risk of sudden infant death syndrome due to swaddling, but this may be linked to other factors. Many generations have used the swaddling technique safely and successfully.

▸ **White noise** – Some babies find noises such as a hairdryer, vacuum cleaner or the 'static' of an untuned radio really comforting. There are various downloads and apps that play white noise, as well as specific white noise baby-calming products. Play these soothing sounds as your babies try to nod off.

▸ **Slings** – Twin slings allow you to carry both babies at the same time or use a single sling if only one baby is unsettled. This enables you to move around and do other things, including playing with or reading to older children.

▶ **Bouncy or swinging chairs** – Some babies love them, others don't, but it's worth a shot. The chairs that swing automatically can be a godsend although they take up a fair chunk of space.

▶ **Keep the babies together** – Your twins have spent their entire lives in very close proximity to each other and then suddenly they're on their own in a big, unfamiliar world. Lying together can be comforting for them.

66 The first night was spent trying to figure out how to sleep in the bed together. In the end I half sat up in bed with one on each side facing me so when they woke up I could just latch them on with one arm without moving too much and hopefully not waking up the other. But it was quite scary and lonely at first as it meant that my boyfriend didn't fit in the bed – I used to phone him if something went wrong. 99

Hanna, mum to Zachary and Noah, 18 months

66 It felt like we didn't get any sleep for two weeks. I can dispel the myth of twins being 'in sync'! We would just get one sorted and then the other would wake up, and whatever tricks we tried to get them in sync they just would not play ball. We were bottle-feeding them and ended up with a one-on-one-off rota constantly through the night. 99

Peter, dad to Thomas and Arthur, 18 months;
and Edward, three

66 When we got home my boyfriend stayed up all night with the babies and I got eight hours' sleep. We worked out a system whereby we both tried to get five hours' sleep. I would go to bed at 11 p.m. and my boyfriend would stay downstairs with

the babies – they were in one Moses basket for the first few weeks and he was on the sofa bed. He would then come up to bed at 4 a.m. and I would do the feeds until 9 a.m. We felt if we could get five hours in a stretch then we could survive. "

Alison, mum to Sylvie and Mila, 12 months

Finding your feet as a family does not happen quickly and the first few weeks will be a cocoon of joy, experimentation, tears, tiredness, immense pride, visitors and gifts of cute matching outfits. A routine will still be a while off (see Chapter 13), but you will start to recognise which part of the day is most stressful, which times are likely to be the most productive and when is a good time for visitors.

You will probably be able to pinpoint more clearly what your needs will be when paternity leave ends and Mummy has to manage by herself. Your other children will also be making their reaction to your twins clear and this has to be factored in, too. As discussed in Chapter 5, hopefully you will have reinforcements waiting in the wings, but you may need to fine-tune your help options now that the babies have arrived.

Tips for the first few weeks at home:

▶ **Don't try to do too much** – Take the pressure off yourself by lowering your expectations and congratulating yourself when you meet them. Getting your babies up, fed and entertained, while keeping the pile of dirty washing down to a small hillock, is no mean feat. If you can get out of the front door, you're into gold-star territory.

▶ **Take this time to get to know your babies as individuals** – When there are (hopefully) plenty of helping hands around. Sometimes it is hard to simply sit and cuddle one baby because you are always conscious that the other one needs you or is missing out.

▶ **Manage your visitors** – Choose times that suit *you* and let your guests look after themselves when they arrive. Having visits from family and friends is a great morale boost, but they are tiring, too, so keep the visits short if you are flagging. If you're having trouble deciding who should visit, ask each guest to bring you a home-cooked dinner. That will sort the wheat from the chaff.

▶ **Enjoy it** – Your babies are super-cute, tiny and a joy to behold. Remember to take loads of photos and label them, especially if your twins are identical. They will never be this small again.

> ❝ I do a 'picture of the day' with a little story which I send to their grandparents. It acts as a diary of sorts and is a good way of stopping and appreciating the girls. ❞
>
> *Gabby, mum to Florrie and Astrid, aged 12 weeks*

Chapter 12

Sleep Deprivation

If you've ever staggered straight into work from an all-night party and thought you'd known what sleep deprivation feels like, this chapter contains some disappointing news. You don't. Yet.

Not for nothing is sleep deprivation intelligence agencies' torture tool of choice. Most new parents will be taken to the limits of their sanity, and in some cases well beyond it, by extreme tiredness as the care of their newborn twins gets under way.

One parent of twins described sleep deprivation as 'a grey feeling, which starts in your tummy and spreads through your body'. You will feel slightly detached and in a bit of a fog; concentration will be difficult and your memory is likely to be poor. Your tolerance of everyday minor irritations suddenly drops and many people find themselves unexpectedly tearful over trivial incidents or, sometimes, nothing at all. The relentless demands of caring for your twins can seem overwhelming and sometimes this tips over into more serious forms of depression, which are covered in further detail in Chapter 14.

As you can't store sleep or prepare for its absence, you may well feel that ignorance is bliss on this topic, but it is worth delving a little into the effects of sleep deprivation, so that when you find yourself sobbing uncontrollably because someone put too much milk in your tea you have some idea why.

66 I think the worst thing about the first six months was definitely the sleep deprivation. When they were about four months old I completely lost the plot one day and my husband found all three of us crying in the rain. He hired a night nanny to come for three nights and sort us out. That was the beginning of routine, which is now our best friend, and she did some very gentle sleep training to get them napping in their cots rather than in the pushchair. It changed our lives, everyone was much happier, and we have never looked back. They are still not amazing sleepers... but we cope. 99

Lindsay, mum to Alex and Serafina, 22 months

66 At one point I kept a notebook by my bed and started obsessively writing down the times (to the minute) that I went to sleep and woke up, and would calculate how much sleep I'd had over a 24-hour period – it was usually about four hours. I was just so tired I think I wanted to try to get some sort of control on the situation and in some ways it did help – it meant I could tell everybody how little sleep I'd had! 99

Pip, mum to Polly and Bertie, two; and Charlie, 12 months

66 I had a cycle of dealing with sleep deprivation – firstly I'd think how unbelievably hard it was, then think that everyone goes through this so surely it must get better and finally think how much worse it would be if I didn't have the babies. Then I'd loop back to thinking how unbelievably hard it was. 99

Ming, dad to Alfred and Joseph, two

Partners often find this period really difficult as they are being very hands-on at home and then having to function at work, too. Concentrating on your job after a night up with the babies is pretty tough and not all employers appreciate just how much extra work is involved when you are a dad of twins. As a couple, it is easy to get competitive over who has had the least sleep and who is having the hardest time.

> ❝ I have to drive for almost an hour to get to work and then back again which after hardly any sleep wasn't fun. I was lucky because my employer was very understanding and if I'd had a night of literally no sleep I didn't go into work that day. I decided not to try to be macho about it and was quite upfront with my boss, which made it a lot easier to deal with and, as a result, people at work were really great. ❞
>
> *Peter, dad to Thomas and Arthur, 18 months;*
> *and Edward, three*

> ❝ I had a job interview when the twins were a week old. I was completely honest with them and told them my life was going to be chaos for a while, but they gave me the job anyway. I lost count of how many times I turned up for work after an hour or two's sleep, sometimes less, and I still had to go in and be professional. Caffeine and sugar became my best friends. But no matter how hard it was, it was still a hell of a lot easier than being with the twins – at least I could have a cup of tea and drink it while it was still hot, which is more than my wife could do at home. ❞
>
> *James, dad to Rosie and Elliott, seven months;*
> *and Robin, three*

The only way to counter sleep deprivation is to sleep, and even a few hours snatched during the day will help. But the standard advice to 'sleep when the babies sleep' is often greeted with a hollow laugh from mothers and fathers of twins. This assumes that your babies sleep at the same time, that you don't have to go off to work and that you don't have other children to look after, too. If you are fortunate enough to get coordinated naps then resist any urge to tidy, cook or check your phone and head straight for bed.

If you have anyone helping you, ask them to take the babies out in the pram once you have fed them so that you have a completely quiet house in which to rest. Listening to your mother-in-law fumbling for nappies in the next room as one or both babies cry is not conducive to a good rest.

In the first few weeks it is very difficult to delegate night-time feeding as you are all finding your way through the process. However, once feeding has become more established and you are able to express milk or are bottle-feeding, it might be possible to take the night feeds in turns. For example, once the babies are fed at, say, 10 p.m., you head straight to bed and let your partner take the next feed. If you are lucky, you might get a three to four-hour stint of sleep and can then take the next feed, enabling your partner to do the same. (See Chapter 13 for more ideas.)

The plus side of having so little sleep is that when you do get more than three hours in a row it feels like a virtual lie-in. You will surprise yourself by how little sleep you can function on and how much better you feel the few times you get just a little bit more continuous shut-eye.

There is no denying, though, that with not enough sleep the constant demands of your babies can occasionally feel overwhelming, particularly if they cry a lot or you are having problems feeding.

Tips to help you if it all gets a bit much:

► Make sure your babies are safely positioned in their cot(s) then leave the room and shut the door. Go somewhere that you cannot hear the crying (downstairs or the garden) or put on some headphones. For five or ten minutes have a cup of tea and breathe deeply. You will be calmer and better able to deal with the situation when you return.

► Do what you have to do. This is not the time to worry about getting into bad habits or your mum's views on dummies. If it is 3 a.m. and you can get your babies to sleep by driving them around the block for ten minutes, pushing them down the road in the buggy or playing Mozart over their cots, then do it.

► It may sound counterintuitive, but if your babies are crying and you are finding it hard to cope, it can help to get them into the buggy and all of you out of the door. Often the movement of the buggy will soothe them and simply being out of the house can make you feel better. If they continue crying, stare straight ahead, don't meet anyone's eye, take deep breaths and give yourself 15 minutes of walking round the block before you return. By then, they may well have fallen asleep.

► Make sure you are eating properly. You will eat plenty of cake and treats, but you also need lots of water, fruit and vegetables to energise your poor, tired body.

❝ We were having a terrible time getting the girls to sleep and as they were suckling on me, but not getting much from it, the midwife suggested trying dummies. We did and it worked really well and we got a bit of sleep at last. The next morning my in-laws came over and saw the dummies in their cot – the guilt of it! The girls had got themselves to the point where they were being sick by crying and these dummies had helped, but there I was considering taking them away just to please my mother-in-law, because I didn't want to be judged. 〞

Emily, mum to Willow and Mia, six weeks

〝 There were definitely a couple of occasions when I had to go into another room. I just needed to not hear the shouting for a minute and refresh myself. For everybody's sake, I stood and smelt the fresh air and prepared myself for round two. 〞

Milly, mum to Alfred and Joseph, two

〝 There were nights when the twins were crying and they'd wake our older son up so he'd come out and want a cuddle. It would be 3 a.m., we were standing in the dark on the landing, each holding a screaming baby and we'd look at each other and think 'How the hell do we do this?'. It was almost hilarious. 〞

James, dad to Rosie and Elliott, seven months; and Robin, three

It may seem hard to believe at the moment, but keep telling yourself that it will get better – it *will* get better. As soon as you start getting even a fraction more sleep, you will feel more like your old self and more able to cope.

Chapter 13

Getting into a Routine

Reaching a stage where your babies not only feed but sleep at roughly the same times each day and every day is, for some lucky parents, the turning point in surviving the first year of raising twins. When this routine extends to a lengthy period of continuous night-time sleep, you have truly found the holy grail.

However, as some mums and dads are luxuriating in five or six hours of uninterrupted sleep, others are mired in almost continuous night-time feeds only to endure difficult days of uncoordinated naptimes and grizzling babies.

If you fall into the semi-comatose camp, it is hard not to feel you are doing something wrong when other parents around you seem to be getting their act together and proclaiming loudly about how much easier life is becoming.

Getting into a routine isn't easy for everyone and it doesn't happen overnight. Often a lot of trial and error is required before you find a system that works for you. The key to establishing good sleep patterns is to set up good feeding patterns, so take one step at a time, get to know your babies, and together your days and nights will start to take shape.

How to set up a routine: feeding and sleeping

A routine should be an ordering of the day that suits you and the babies, loosely based on their natural sleep patterns. It doesn't have to mean adopting a rigid timetable whereby every second of the day is mapped out, including when to open the curtains and what to give yourself for breakfast. Some people find that level of detail reassuring and like having a clear set of instructions to follow, while others find the whole idea of a routine restrictive and prefer to respond to the needs of their individual babies.

Many parents of twins settle on a system somewhere in the middle – a routine that gives everybody a bit of wriggle room, but allows the babies to have clear and predictable meal and naptimes.

That's all very well in principle, but how on earth do you persuade two babies to do the same thing at the same time? The honest answer is that sometimes you can't, but all babies need to sleep and eat, and these are the two central tenets of any routine. Consider this your first lesson in the gentle art of parental manipulation.

As we have already heard, the majority of twins are born prematurely and even those who go to term tend to have smaller birth weights than single babies. Small babies need lots of feeding on demand when they first come home and it is not realistic to expect to get them into a routine for at least three weeks, possibly considerably longer depending on their health and weight. The smaller or more poorly the baby, the longer it may take, although premature babies who have spent time in special care will usually leave hospital with a feeding routine in place. Initially, concentrate on feeding your babies when they need it, establishing your milk supply or getting your bottle-feeding system in place, and focus on increasing their weight.

Once your babies are being fed about every three to four hours, you will probably start to develop a mini routine. Feeds often start around 7 a.m., then follow at mid-morning, lunchtime, mid-afternoon and then around 6.30–7 p.m. just before bedtime. Night feeds will continue at roughly the same intervals. As your babies get bigger and stronger and can go longer between feeds, you will gradually drop the 10 p.m. feed and, with luck, start to push back the 1–2 a.m. feed to achieve the jackpot: sleeping through the night.

One of the keys to establishing good sleep patterns is to avoid excessive 'snacking' and comfort sucking, and instead encourage good feeds at every session. This can be difficult with sleepy babies who often nod off as soon as they start feeding. Methods of keeping them awake, such as tickling their feet or rubbing their back, are extremely comforting, but they can be so enjoyable that they lull your babies right back to sleep. A gentle way of waking them up properly for a feed is to change their nappies beforehand, regardless of whether it is necessary or not.

Lots of parents find it helpful to keep a note of sleep times and feeds in the early days. This allows you to keep track of who's been fed and how much they've taken or, in breastfeeding terms, of how long they've been feeding. If one baby is sleeping less well, it may be because they are not taking enough milk at feeding time – or that they require extra – and your notes will help you work out any adjustments that need to be made.

Most routines follow the basic idea of encouraging predictable periods of sleep, naps and awake or 'play' time. Initially, naptimes often fall quite naturally first thing in the morning (about an hour and a half to two hours after waking), around lunchtime and then again in mid to late afternoon. Some parents panic that if their babies sleep too much during the day they won't sleep at night, but newborn babies need a lot of sleep (anything from eight to 18 hours a day) and regular naps can help them sleep better at night. Some babies become overtired and are extremely hard to settle as a result of limited daytime sleeps.

Everyone has their own approach to naps. Some parents will not wake their sleeping babies; others will wake them at set times because they are worried that too much sleep in one session will mean they sleep less well at the next. Unless you want to follow a pre-planned routine, such as Gina Ford's schedule, you will need to experiment a little with sleep times. As the first year progresses, the late-afternoon nap may drop off and the early-morning nap may shorten. By the time your twins are between 12 and 18 months, the lunchtime nap will become their only daytime sleep.

66 I thought we would just go freestyle and not do any schedules but it just couldn't happen. Initially the boys had to be fed every three hours so there was no way of dealing with that apart from being super organised. When we were able to relax that routine we tried to do it our way but it was complete mayhem! We went back to a lesser routine but tried to do it slightly more flexibly, with a basic 'eat, sleep and play' structure. 99

Milly, mum to Alfred and Joseph, two

66 I am not a particularly organised person in my own life, but I am heavily into a routine with the children. In the early days I kept getting to classes and finding they were asleep. I didn't really want to be sitting there singing silly songs when the babies were fast asleep – in the end I found life was more relaxed if I knew what was going to happen. I followed Gina Ford, but pretty loosely. It worked for us.

They were good sleepers and then at about three months they'd be fine all day but at about 7 p.m. they'd start wailing. We tried everything, including walking them round the block, but nothing worked and we had three weeks of horrific evenings; and then one day it just stopped. 99

Katie, mum to Keira and Gracie, 11 months; and Layla, five

66 Nell was three and about to start nursery when Alex and Jake were born so I needed to be on the ball. We were really, really lucky because the boys had good birth weights and were very sleepy babies, so right from day one we woke

them every four hours so I could breastfeed them at the same time. I would feed them and never let them fall asleep 'on the boob'. When I had Nell I never thought I'd ever be a campaigner for routine, but with the twins, this was one thing I felt I had control over! 〝

Sarah, mum to Alex and Jake, six; and Nell, nine

Many parents worry that their twins will disturb and wake each other up, so can be quick to pick up a crying baby. Often, however, the sleeping baby will be completely oblivious to the racket its brother or sister is making. Keeping the babies together, either in the same cot or the same room, can be comforting to the babies and can help them to settle.

〝I always did a bath, then story, then in bed by 6.30 p.m. They were always really good sleepers and settled really well. They slept through from about 12 weeks. If one cried, I'd pick him up and soothe him and then put him straight down again. I never rocked them to sleep. At first they shared a Moses basket, but by eight weeks they had got too big so we put them in separate cots. I was a bit concerned that they were not going to settle but they were fine – we put their cots across the room so they could see each other and know they were there. Even now, they never come out of their room once we've put them to bed, they have a chat and sometimes they get into each other's bed but they never come out. 〝

Gillian, mum to Benjamin and Finlay, three;
and Joseph, five

> ❝ For me, the key to them sleeping was keeping them together. They shared a cot from when they were in hospital and I won't separate them until they are ready. My husband put two cots together and even today they sleep together in one gigantic cot. ❞
>
> *Clare, mum to Henley and Riley, 19 months; Lexi, three; and Kaysie, nine*

How to set up a routine: bath time and bedtime

Having a defined bedtime is a key component of retaining your sanity in the first year. And it's quite good for the babies, too. Your twins may not sleep at the allotted time, of course, and could well grizzle for several hours before you hit that magic hour, usually around 6–7 p.m., but without a defined bedtime your afternoon will drag into your evening, and before you know it you've had another cold dinner with a baby on your knee and it's time for the next feed.

The period from about 4–6 p.m. can be the hardest of the day, especially if you are by yourself and have other children to care for, too. Naps are over and a combination of hunger and tiredness can make everyone really grumpy.

Many parents have bath time as a central part of their bedtime routine, but bathing baby twins can be very stressful and not all parents feel confident in doing this by themselves. It is perfectly possible to have a calm bedtime routine that does not involve having a bath. You do not need to bath your twins every day and can keep them just as clean with a thorough wash on their changing mat, using water and cotton wool.

Bath-time tips:

▶ Never leave your baby unattended in the bath, even for a second.

▶ Bath one twin at a time when they are small babies. It makes it less stressful for you and is much safer. Alternatively, you could bath one baby one day, and the other baby the following day.

▶ Have everything ready before you start. You will need towels, nappies and cotton pads for washing the babies, as well as clean bedtime outfits.

▶ If you can fit them in your bathroom, have your twins in bouncy chairs or lying on a towel. If not, keep the door open and have them in chairs just outside. If you have an older child, he or she could help by singing to the twin outside the door or by making little waves in the bath.

▶ Make sure the bathroom is nice and warm as babies lose their body heat quickly when naked. Do not undress a baby until everything is ready.

▶ Run the bath using cold water first and top up with hot. Fill to a depth of between 8–10 cm. Check the bathwater temperature using your elbow. It should feel the same as your body temperature – warm, not hot.

▶ You do not need any bubble bath or shampoo – plain water is best for newborn babies.

▶ 'Top and tail' your babies (washing their face, neck, hands and bottom) before putting them in the bath: lay the baby on its towel and use cotton wool pads dipped in the bath water.

▶ Have a firm grip on your baby as you lift them out of the bath, as they will be really slippery.

▶ Dry your babies carefully and thoroughly.

> 66 Until the girls could support themselves in moulded plastic supports, bath time was strictly a two-person job. Slippery babies and porcelain tiles make for dangerous situations. 99
>
> *Sabreena, mum to Yasmin and Nadia, seven*

Parents with older children often find the bath and putting-to-bed period especially hard and may struggle with dividing themselves between three or four tired children who want baths, bottles and bedtime stories at exactly the same time. Be kind to yourself – you can only do your best. If your older children are happy to watch a bit of television, listen to an audiobook or play a game on the iPad, then don't beat yourself up about it and enjoy the time it gives you with your twins.

> 66 My husband often works in the evening so I was regularly having to put everyone to bed, which I found difficult. In the end, I'd put the twins in the carrier – one on my back and one on my front, and I'd read the older two their bedtime stories. Usually the twins fell asleep like that and it did work. 99
>
> *Laura, mum to Rory and Heidi, ten months; Lewis, three; and Niamh, five*

> 66 At bedtime I was putting Ti-Jean to bed first, but then I'd have to feed Maui and Loki, and would spend so much time getting them sorted out that I'd be falling asleep over them. After eight months I was ragged. A friend paid for us to have some sleep training. A woman helped us get into a routine –

central to which was that when they go to bed at night it is important to leave them, you pat them to sleep. It was very gentle. It worked wonders. Had I known that could be done I'd have done it earlier. 🙶

Adwoa, mum to Ti-Jean, six; Maui and Loki, two

🙶I used to dread bedtime. I tried reading to my two year old and getting him to bed and then feeding the twins, but they'd cry all through his storytime and ruin it. But if I fed them first, then I'd have to plonk Rhys in front of the telly while I did it, which I hated, and often they'd still cry through his bedtime anyway. It was really, really hard. 🙶

Mandie, mum to Zadie and Lara, two; and Rhys, four

When it doesn't work

Sometimes, despite patience, experimentation and determination on your part, your babies have their own views about when – or if – they want to sleep and will stubbornly stick to them. You may have to rethink your approach.

Some parents spend a week writing a sleep diary (for the babies, that is – your own sleep diary probably won't take up much ink) to help them work out some natural patterns around which to build a mini-schedule. Others find that once their babies mature to the weaning stage, it becomes easier to set up a routine. Or maybe a routine just isn't for you.

Some families try their own form of sleep training, which involves breaking certain habits at bedtime and encouraging the babies to sleep without parental props, such as rocking or being held. Some opt for the 'gradual retreat', whereby the parent gradually withdraws, perhaps first by putting the babies in the cot and patting them, then sitting by the cot and finally leaving the room completely. A different approach called 'cry it out' suggests leaving babies to cry for short periods, before a parent returns to reassure them and then withdraws once more.

Even if you do successfully get a routine in place, it can be unexpectedly knocked off track by teething, growth spurts or illness. Lots of parents find that they have periods of unsettled evenings for no apparent reason, which often go away just as suddenly, leaving them with no real idea of their cause. Going to stay with friends or relatives or taking a holiday can also disrupt your routine for a while. Having achieved a regular routine once, you can be fairly confident that you can return to it once you get back to 'normal'.

&&Our routine happened quite naturally at about eight months. After weaning they just seemed to find their own routine. Until that point I had been happy with them sleeping in the buggy or wherever, but now I am more conscious of building our day around their routine as I know they sleep better in their cots. 99

Jayne, mum to Thomas and Holly, 11 months

&&The girls were never good sleepers. We had nine months of very little sleep, by which time we were ready to jump. Someone had suggested a system called 'cry it out' which we'd read about for a while, but hadn't wanted to try yet. One day we just decided to do it. I think the hardest thing in the world as a parent was walking out of the room on that first night. They were used to us staying in the room until they fell asleep, but we just couldn't keep going like that. We were dreading hours of crying, but after an hour they had both dropped off and, for the first time ever, they slept through until 6 a.m. It took about two months to get it right, but they've been brilliant ever since. People say they could never do it, but until you're in that position you can't say. **"**

Daniel, dad to Sophie and Hannah, three

" There are positives for no set sleep times, I get lots of quality individual time. It also means when I'm out I don't get so stressed thinking they will both wake at the same time for a feed – I can hold one and then generally swap. Although we do have feed times generally at the same time, when they were small I used to use a dummy to pacify one and then feed separately. Now I feed together if they are both desperate although I prefer to feed one after another. I find it hard to implement a daytime sleep routine as they are so different and I can't force Lola to sleep and I'm not sure I should – I would hate to be told when to sleep. **"**

Sally, mum to Lola and Franklin, six months

Trying to predict whether or not your babies are going to sleep each day becomes something of an obsession when rest of any kind is in short supply – for both you and your children.

Good naps set you all up with more energy, better moods and the ability to cope with the demands of the day. Having a small amount of 'time out' every day at naptime will help you to appreciate your babies and enjoy more of the time you spend together. So if your house is a nap-free zone it may be time to consider more drastic measures, such as employing a sleep consultant or using some sleep-training techniques.

Calling in the professionals

Parents are often very reluctant to call in sleep consultants for fear that a grim-faced matron will descend on their home, whisk their beloved babies into a darkened room, hand them each a pair of earplugs and order them to stop fussing. In fact, sleep consultants are very sensitive to the distress all mums and dads feel when their babies cry and they will try to work out a strategy that reflects your parental philosophy.

Parents need to accept that, even with a delicate approach, the babies are likely to resist a change to their regime, and that their resistance may be painful to listen to. In weighing up whether this is pain you can bear, ask yourself the following questions:

▶ When was the last time I had enough sleep?

▶ Can I carry on like this?

▶ Am I enjoying my babies?

▶ Are my babies happy?

If you feel at the end of your tether and have sufficient funds in the bank, this may be the time to approach a sleep consultant for some advice. Most sleep consultants advertise privately and can be found online, but you may find better recommendations using your local twins club or parents' forum.

66 When you are exhausted it is hard to see the wood for the trees. Everyone starts giving advice about what you should do and you are so desperate you will try lots of things and start to lose your gut instinct about what to do.

If a family contacts me with sleep issues I would look to eliminate feeding issues first, then discomfort, such as reflux, and finally, habit.

In terms of establishing a routine, it's not about the time on the clock, it is the sequence of events. Most of us lead quite routine-based lives and we seem to find quite a lot of security in that. Little people like to know what they are doing, too.

It is really important that Mum gets a break, which is why with twins I recommend introducing one bottle a day of either formula or breast milk by three weeks, assuming the babies are term and healthy, a bit later for early twins. This then allows other people to support Mum at feeding time, which is crucial.

If your babies are not taking enough calories during the day they will make up for it at night. I look for ways of adjusting feeding to get them to take all their calories during the day.

I would expect term, six-week-old babies, with no health problems and who are consistently gaining weight, to start to do a stretch of about five hours a night. Parents of preemie twins need to adjust their expectations of when their babies are strong enough to start to get into a routine. If your eight-week-old babies were four weeks early then you need to think of them as if they are four weeks old.

I talk parents through the different sleep-training methods. If parents are against controlled crying, I would work through the idea of gradual retreat. It depends what the parents want to try and it is important that the method feels manageable as they will then be able to stick to it. Parents choose the method, but there is always a period of resistance and it can be stressful, but how long has this family been sleep deprived for?

A lot of parents don't admit to anyone that they are using my services because they are so scared that they are going to be judged. If only we could all be a bit kinder and a bit more accepting of peoples' choices – we are all trying our best and when it does go wrong the last thing we need is for other people to point it out to us. We feel bad enough already!

Parents usually come to me exhausted and not believing it will work, so when it does, it's wonderful. 🙶

Annie Simpson, infant sleep consultant

Don't despair

As all new parents know, sleep deprivation is hard enough to bear for a few weeks, let alone for months or, in some cases, years. Don't suffer alone if you are not getting enough sleep. If you can't afford sleep-training advice, visit online forums or try to link up with a local postnatal or twins group for some support and practical help.

Small changes in approach can make big differences to the effectiveness of your routine. Ask one trusted, supportive friend or relative to help you take a step back and look at your day objectively. Discuss your observations and make some tweaks based on what you discover.

Some babies really do sleep more than others and if a routine is proving elusive then you are simply unlucky, not a failure. Don't give up. Most babies do eventually find their sleep groove. Do what you have to do to get through the bad nights and be kind to yourself during the day. Enlist as much help as you can to keep your sleep topped up to minimum levels.

As unlikely as it may feel, you will get through this. Keep putting one foot in front of the other and you will reach all those happy times that lie ahead.

Chapter 14

Postnatal Depression

New parents of twins are often exhausted, over emotional, weepy or anxious. In amongst all these feelings, there is a fair dollop of joy, pride, laughter and happiness. Postnatal depression throws a black cloak over all of those positive emotions. It steals your confidence; it deprives you of even the basic energy you need to get up in the morning; it transforms everyday tasks into terrifying ordeals; and robs you of your belief that you will ever get through this illness. At its worst, it may even temporarily dim the love you have for your babies.

It is thought that about one in ten new mothers experience PND, but a survey by the Twins and Multiple Birth Association found that 26 per cent of mothers of twins or triplets believed they might have suffered from PND, with 13 per cent 'sure' they had and the same number 'not sure'. With the additional strains of caring for two new babies, perhaps it shouldn't be a surprise that mothers of twins are more likely to be susceptible to this illness.

Postnatal depression is a serious mental illness and must be treated. This usually, but not always, involves taking antidepressants combined with forms of talking therapies. Many women suffering from PND find that talking to others who have been through the same experience via local support groups or online forums helps them to start to believe that recovery is possible.

What causes PND?

There are many factors involved in this condition but it can affect anyone, even if you've never had any depression before. If you have recently experienced other life-changing events in addition to having your twins, such as an illness or death in the family, a break-up of a relationship, losing your job or moving house, this can also increase the likelihood of PND. Mothers lacking support – particularly young, single mums – are more vulnerable. Women who have suffered from depression or mental health problems before their pregnancy are more susceptible to PND, so it is important to talk through coping mechanisms with health professionals before the birth of your twins.

However, sometimes there are no obvious warning signs and PND can strike quickly and debilitatingly, taking everyone in your circle of family and friends by surprise.

Recognising postnatal depression

It is extremely common to suffer from 'baby blues' about three to ten days after giving birth, which will make you feel weepy and emotional, often at unexpected times or out of nowhere. However, this feeling is manageable and passes quickly.

Postnatal depression is something else altogether. It is persistent, all encompassing and does not go away. It usually strikes within six weeks of giving birth, although it can develop at any time during the first year after birth. Sometimes its effects are felt gradually but it can also be very sudden.

66 Everyone feels tired after having a baby, particularly when you have twins, but the signs to look out for are feeling that you are not enjoying your babies, wanting to be left alone, not wanting to engage with other people and feeling emotional and tearful. 99

Dr Saima Latif, chartered psychologist, mum to Faris and Haris, seven

Symptoms and signs of postnatal depression:

▶ Feeling sad and low

▶ Being tearful

▶ Feeling worthless

▶ Panic attacks

▶ Feeling hopeless

▶ Tiredness

▶ Feeling irritable and angry

▶ Feeling guilty

▶ Feeling hostile or indifferent to either your partner or babies

▶ Loss of concentration

▶ Finding it hard to sleep – even when you get the chance

▶ Lack of appetite

▶ Unwillingness to see people or to go out

▶ Thoughts about death

❝ I had absolutely no depression at all before this. I had one cry with my first baby at three days and nothing for my second. I even have a background in mental health rehabilitation, so I went from being the professional to the client, which is something that had never crossed my mind would happen.

I had quite an isolated beginning of my pregnancy with the girls. I am a single parent to my two boys and my relationship with the girls' dad was not that long established, so I was living on my own with the boys at that point. I had had a very easy first pregnancy, but now with this one everything seemed to be high risk and there was a lack of personal care as a result. It felt as if I was being passed from consultant to consultant and there was no continuity, nobody to notice if there was any emotional instability. It seemed like I had very little control in this pregnancy — I kept my head down and concentrated on growing the twins, but there was nothing for me.

The twins were born by C-section and I was obsessed by how many people were in the operating theatre. When it got to 20 I said I needed to know how many were there as it seemed to be the only thing I had any control over. It wasn't necessary to be that anxious, but I couldn't see that. After they were born I had one baby in special care and one baby with me, and it completely threw me, as I was unprepared for them to be split up. I had imagined we'd all be together and I found it hard to get through to my brain what had happened.

It was my birthday two days after I got home from hospital and from then on I was in this postnatal-depression bubble. I was lucky that it never affected the way I felt about the children, but I found it really hard to function for myself. I'd wake up in the morning and have to ask my partner how to get ready.

I was lucky because the health visitor spotted signs of PND quickly and I got 13 sessions with a psychologist on the NHS who was brilliant, I am also on medication, even now.

It had a huge effect on our lives though. My partner lost his job as he had to be the main carer, and I was in a dark place for a long time. It felt like the only thing I wanted to do was take a bag of medication, go into the woods and go to sleep. I felt emotionally so exhausted I couldn't think how I could let my brain rest. I tried to visualise what would happen and kept telling myself that I wouldn't see my children get married if I went through with it. I have had panic attacks where complete strangers have had to help me and had situations where people I didn't know stopped their cars and offered to help me because I was standing with the children in floods of tears. I wouldn't have wanted it to happen, but I have experienced so much human kindness.

I've been really lucky in that there is a great, free local support group for depression run by one of the dads at school. I don't even go that much, but just to know it's there helps me. I've been quite open about having PND and so many mothers have told me that they have had PND, too – it is so common, but people don't talk about it because they think they'll be judged. There are so many organisations out there that can help, it's really important to tell people how you're feeling. 99

Janine, mum to Wren and Taryn, 19 months; Jaden, ten; and Morten, 12

Getting help

Despite far greater awareness of the seriousness of PND, many women are still very reluctant to acknowledge that they are suffering from depression or to get help. Mothers of twins sometimes assume that their symptoms are 'normal' because looking after twins will make you feel doubly tired or low. Some mothers are terrified that their babies will be taken away from them if they are found to have PND and are reluctant to ask for help from professionals as a result. Others assume that they can't be experiencing PND because they've never had mental health problems in the past and have had a good, happy pregnancy.

Your health visitor should be looking for signs of PND as routine and may ask you to fill in a questionnaire asking how you feel. Sometimes mums find it easier to answer this questionnaire honestly rather than actually asking for help. However, not all health visitors pick up on signs of PND and it may be partners or families who realise that something is wrong and then try to persuade you to see your GP.

Getting better

The sooner PND is diagnosed, the quicker it can be treated. Although mothers who have seen themselves alter so dramatically as a result of this condition often feel pessimistic about the chances of returning to their 'old selves', a full recovery is absolutely possible – but it will take time and involve changes at home to help you get better.

You should be offered professional help in the form of talking therapies, such as psychotherapy or counselling, and, depending on the severity of your PND, antidepressants may be prescribed, too. These often have side effects, which will be discussed, and may impact on your ability to breastfeed.

> Antidepressants do help for a short time and can be useful for getting you back on an even keel. Mothers are worried that they will get addicted to them or won't ever be able to cope without them, but for a short time they can stabilise your mood. Therapy is also useful as it gives you the toolkit to manage difficulties and show you how to cope in situations that you may have found overwhelming.
>
> Many women despair that they will ever recover from postnatal depression, but it has to be thought of as a repairable injury. If you broke your leg and the doctor who put a cast on it told you you'd always be like that, you wouldn't

believe him. It's the same for a mental injury – you're not going to be like that for the rest of your life. With help, you will get better. "

Dr Saima Latif, chartered psychologist, and mum to Faris and Haris, seven

As well as professional help, you and those supporting you can make changes at home to help your recovery.

Changes to consider making if you suffer from PND:

▶ **Diet** – Although you may well have a very small appetite, eating healthy foods and drinking plenty of water are really important to your body's recovery.

▶ **Exercise** – You may feel that getting out is almost impossible and that exercise is the last thing you want to do, but exercise can help you start to feel better. If you are able to get someone to sit with the babies for an hour, ask a friend to come along to an exercise class with you or you could simply walk round the block together.

▶ **Meet other mums** – Almost all women who have suffered from PND say that the encouragement of other mothers in the same position gave them belief in their own recovery. Your GP may be able to recommend a local support group and there are lots of excellent online support groups, too.

▶ **Let go** – Many women seem programmed to put everyone else's needs before their own, even when they are seriously ill. To recover from PND, you need rest and to get this with newborn twins requires a lot of help, either from family, friends or someone who is paid. Anything that is not essential, such as housework, should be put to one side and all priority given to your rest and recovery.

> ❝I had no history of depression at all, in fact I remember watching a programme about having babies and thinking that at least postnatal depression was something I didn't need to worry about.
>
> My pregnancy was quite difficult, but mentally I was really well. Because of the boys' positions I had an elective caesarean, which was very straightforward. Being in hospital was hard as I couldn't really stand up and had to look after two babies, but I remember experiencing the baby blues and being a bit weepy, and then it passing and going away again, as I was expecting.
>
> I had very severe stomach pain after the caesarean which just didn't go away. I couldn't lift the boys and it was very difficult to look after them. The doctors were convinced that I had an infection so put me on high doses of antibiotics, which didn't seem to do anything, eventually putting me on ones which meant I couldn't breastfeed the boys any more and I think that had a really big impact. About six weeks afterwards I had a massive, massive panic attack. Because I wasn't breastfeeding I had a very early period and I think the combination of hormones, antibiotics and their side effects, being in pain and having the twins left me in a very bad way. Eventually I was taken to hospital and they discovered that I had a hernia, so the antibiotics were never even needed.
>
> By then I was having almost constant panic attacks. They felt like somebody was holding a gun to my head except there's nobody there and there's no gun. I couldn't see a way out and was absolutely terrified. I had always been a practical, down-

to-earth, independent and completely with-it person and now I couldn't open the door, couldn't leave the house. I couldn't imagine that I could ever get better. I couldn't remember what it felt like to be the person I was beforehand.

The one thing that I was thankful for was that I never lost my connection with the boys. My mum came to help and my husband was very hands on, but I always cared for them and loved them, and I know that isn't always the case with depression. But I was so far removed from the person I had been that I felt I was going through the motions – every task, like getting out the pram to walk to the shops to get nappies, felt like a huge mountain to climb. I couldn't make any plans. The world seemed to shrink and everything needed minute-to-minute planning, otherwise I couldn't do it. It was almost as if I needed nannying – sometimes if my husband was working at night, my dad would come over and sit with me because I couldn't bear to be alone.

My husband found it impossible because he just couldn't understand what had happened to me. I'd always spent quite a lot of time on my own and been independent, and then I just couldn't be on my own – I was terrified. He got very angry about it at times and with me because he couldn't understand. I was so unlike myself that my family didn't know what they were dealing with.

The really horrendous period lasted for about six months and I slowly started to come out of it. I think it was a combination of medication, seeing a psychologist, and talking and reading about people who'd been through the same thing and come out the other side. I went to a postnatal support group led by someone who had suffered from postnatal depression twice. I kept thinking of her and feeling that she'd managed to come through it and that gave me hope that I could.

The boys were born in April and I went back to work the following January, but I'd say it took a good couple of years to fully recover. The depression completely rocked my confidence, because I'd always thought I could deal with anything and this made me realise that I couldn't. I have had a few small recurrences since and I don't think I could ever say that it won't return, but it's not something that I see as a weakness or something to be worried about now. 〞

Sally, mum to Jack and Luke, 15

Being diagnosed with postnatal depression can be a frightening and shocking experience, but it is also the starting point of your recovery. Reaching out to the people around you by acknowledging your struggle with this condition is a difficult and courageous decision. By doing so, you will hopefully find the support, treatment and understanding you need to throw off the black cloak of depression and return to the sunshine to enjoy your babies. (See the Resources and Further Reading chapter for suggestions on where to turn if you think you may be suffering from PND.)

Chapter 15

Getting Out and About

Opening the front door and leaving the house should be one of life's more straightforward tasks, but when you add the risk of stereo shrieking, the probability of a double bottom explosion and the paparazzi-style attention of the general public, getting out and about with your twins can seem like a monumental effort.

For the first few weeks you may go into semi-hibernation while you all find your feet as a family, but at some point the art of getting out of the house with two small babies has to be mastered.

Gone, for now, are impromptu lunches and quick dashes to the shops for a pint of milk. You'll still go to the shop for a pint of milk, of course, but it is unlikely to be at a dash, trot or anything exceeding a painfully slow crawl. Cafes are no longer judged on the quality of their coffee but on the square footage of their premises. A visit to somewhere new requires a detailed reconnaissance and military planning.

Watching friends with single babies breeze off to tiny, trendy cafes for lunch or hearing about their one-to-one bonding at tots swimming classes can be really irritating when you have worn yourself out simply trying to get your twins as far as the front door. It can't be denied that your life is slightly more complicated than theirs at the moment, but that doesn't mean it isn't without just as many special moments.

How to actually get out of the house
As we've established, getting out of the house with tiny twins *is* a big deal. Your timetable may look something like this:

9 a.m.	Stock changing bag with nappies, wipes, vests, Babygros and muslin squares
9.05 a.m.	Break off to change first baby's nappy
9.10 a.m.	Resume filling changing bag
9.13 a.m.	Break off to wipe sick off second baby
9.16 a.m.	Finish filling changing bag, but will six changes of clothes be enough?
9.20 a.m.	Stash extra baby clothes underneath the buggy
9.25 a.m.	Prepare bag of emergency feeding options
9.30 a.m.	Break off to pick up crying baby
9.35 a.m.	Rock second crying baby with foot as first baby continues to howl
9.40 a.m.	Put buggy in position by the door
9.42 a.m.	Wrestle first baby into outdoor gear. Does he need a hat?
9.45 a.m.	Find hat
9.46 a.m.	Pick hat off the floor and jam it back on baby's head
9.48 a.m.	Put second baby into outdoor gear and strap into the buggy
9.50 a.m.	Retrieve two hats from the floor and put them back in the cupboard
9.52 a.m.	Go to the toilet
9.55 a.m.	Open the door and leave the house
9.57 a.m.	Stop to tell a stranger: 'Yes, they are twins. But, no, they're not identical.'
9.59 a.m.	Reply to the inevitable comment: 'Yes! My hands are full!'
10.02 a.m.	Arrive at the corner shop
10.03 a.m.	Buy a loaf of bread
10.10 a.m.	Return home

Whether your destination is Mount Kilimanjaro or your local playgroup, it is impossible to leave the house without groaning under the weight of bags of spare clothes, equipment and food. No matter how well organised you are, unexpected interruptions are inevitable and punctuality becomes, frankly, a rather overrated quality. Just add this to the growing list of items from which control is slipping.

Getting from A to B (without going via Z)

If you are going further afield, careful planning is required so that you don't find yourself stranded with your double buggy at the bottom of an escalator or facing a vertiginous set of stairs alone.

A few things to double check before you visit somewhere new:

▸ Is there parking nearby, preferably family-friendly with extra space to unload?

▸ Are there any lifts? If not, is there any alternative to using stairs (i.e. ramps)?

▸ Are there any family-friendly toilets/baby-change areas big enough to fit a double buggy inside?

▸ Is the cafe big enough to fit a double buggy?

▸ Are there plenty of high chairs?

▸ If you are visiting with an older sibling, is there anywhere enclosed (play area, cafe section with toys), for peace of mind while you eat or snack?

Travelling by public transport can be stressful and, no matter how much you prepare, there is much more chance of your carefully laid plans going awry thanks to breakdowns, lateness or overcrowding.

A few tips for travelling by public transport:

▶ Getting on buses with a double buggy is not easy, although it has become a lot better since many modern vehicles have wheelchair (and therefore buggy) friendly low floors. If there is a double middle door the driver will usually let you board there, once passengers have got off. Often there is a limit to how many buggies are allowed on at one time, so sometimes the driver won't let you on, even if the bus is otherwise relatively quiet.

▶ If you travel by bus regularly, it may be easier to use a single buggy and a sling while the babies are small.

▶ Always wheel the buggy off buses or trains backwards (you first, then the buggy) so that there's no risk of your babies toppling out.

▶ Check access to train stations, as they often involve stairs. Phone the station to double check that lifts are working.

▶ Don't be afraid to ask for help, either from staff or fellow passengers, if you meet an unexpected obstacle.

> 66 To go out I'd take one baby to the car, come back for the second, come back for Joseph and then come back for my bags. Then I'd have to do it all again at the other end! I'd get them all into the pram and then only walk a short distance to playgroup. With one baby you'd just carry it, but it's impossible with twins. Everything was such hard work! Because I had Joseph I got out and about every day, it was almost harder work to stay at home. At least when we went out to a play centre, Joseph was being entertained. 99
>
> *Gillian, mum to Benjamin and Finlay, three; and Joseph, five*

Getting out there

Sooner or later life has to go on, which means resuming shopping, getting out to see friends, visiting parks and playgroups, and generally facing the outside world.

You will find that it has changed since you last ventured out. Doorways seem that bit smaller, pavements a little narrower and everything seems to take so much longer than it did before the babies arrived.

You will rapidly whittle down your excursions and shopping options based on proximity, convenience and automatic doors. Enormous covered shopping malls may not have been your hangout of choice pre-twins, but with their handy parking, expansive baby-change suites and wide walkways you may soon come to see them as a godsend when you feel ready to face shopping again.

> My local supermarket only had two trolleys with two baby seats on them and they kept them inside the store by the information desk. To get one, you had to turn up really early, preferably on a Monday or else they'd be gone. I'd have to wheel the buggy into the supermarket, grab a double trolley, transfer the babies into the trolley and then wheel the buggy and trolley back to the car to get rid of the buggy. It didn't take long to switch to Internet shopping.

Kelly, mum to Shakira and Surai, three

> Everyone kept telling me to do Internet food shopping, but if I had a spare 30 minutes in the evening, the last thing I wanted to do was to spend it doing shopping. So I still go to Tesco, but the twins nearly always fall asleep in the car and I'm too

terrified of waking them up to transfer them to the trolley, so I push the trolley with one hand, and the buggy with the other! Everyone knows us in there. I sometimes have to take the four of them in with me. People need to eat and I need wine so I have to do it! 🙶

Laura, mum to Heidi and Rory, ten months; Lewis, three; and Niamh, five

Committing to a few regular activities motivates you to get out, whether that's to a playgroup, a weekly lunch with a friend or a walk around your local park. Often the alternative – another housebound day with only baby babbling for conversation – acts as a spur.

🙶 Making sure you get out of the house every day is really important for both the mental health of the carer and the health of the children. Who wants to be stuck in the house with babies that won't settle? Exercise and social contact can really help counter feelings of isolation – even if that is just a two-minute conversation at the checkout at Sainsbury's. If you're a single carer with twins, having a stranger stop and say how lovely your babies are is really, really valuable. 🙶

Dr Sarah Helps, consultant clinical psychologist and family therapist, and mum to 12-year-old twins

If you have a twins club near you (you can find your nearest one through the Twins and Multiple Birth Association or contact your local authority), make this your number one priority for the week. Here you will find a fellowship of equally harassed, disorganised and dazed parents who will think nothing of the fact that you've turned up with your jumper on inside out ten minutes before the session finishes. The solidarity that a good twins club offers far outweighs the effort of getting yourselves there. Hopefully you will forge lasting friendships and enjoy a few hours of feeling 'normal' in the company of like-minded mums and dads. It is also a brilliant place to get ideas for things to do and swap parenting advice.

> 66 The first time we went to our twins club, some children shot past us and I could hear someone inside saying, 'You grab those, I've got yours.' That's how it was, we all understood that two kids was too much and just looked after each other. If a kid was crying, you picked it up and everyone was the same. We made so many friends there and we're still great friends with the families of three sets of twins from that group. 99
>
> ***Darren, dad to Mattie and Evie, ten; and Eliza, three***

Showstoppers

Baby twins have a habit of attracting attention. It may be their super-cuteness or the fact that their buggy takes up most of the pavement. Either way, people find them impossible to ignore. This can be lovely and no one enjoys basking in the glory of their own children more than new parents, but it is also time consuming and, after a while, extremely repetitive.

On good days, the comments of strangers can give you a boost and remind you how lucky you are to have twins, but on bad days they can feel rude, intrusive and infuriatingly ignorant. Parents whose twins were conceived by IVF may find casual questions about their conception particularly offensive. It would probably be easier to cope with the public's attention if everyone didn't say exactly the same thing.

A taster of comments you're likely to hear when you're out and about with your twins:

1. **Are they twins?** Let's see… Two similarly sized babies being pushed by an exhausted-looking woman who still looks five months pregnant. That would probably be a yes.

2. **You've got your hands full!** Darned right, but if you could use one of your spare ones to open that door, I'd be really happy. Some American mums like to respond with a cheery 'Just imagine how full my heart is!' Tried on a British audience, this has a satisfyingly nauseating effect.

3. **Are they identical?** This will be asked regardless of whether your children are different sizes, have different hair colour or are lying under pink and blue blankets. Parents of boy/girl twins find it understandably infuriating. Sometimes a 'no' has to be followed up with an explanatory biological update.

4. **Are they natural?** The subtext is clear, but you can choose to ignore it. A deadpan 'No, they're plasticine' can deter further interrogation. Strangers may find it perfectly acceptable to ask about the conception of your twins. You, however, have the option of ignoring their question, giving a misleading answer or asking them why they feel this is any of their business.

5. **Rather you than me.** Can't argue with that, mate.

6 **Ooh, double trouble!** If you're feeling kind, you could reply: 'Yes, but double the fun, too.' This may or may not be true at this particular moment in time.

7 **Who is older?** If you pause on this one, the questioner will almost certainly try to guess. Why it is of interest to a stranger is a mystery. But it is.

8 **Who is the naughty one?** Perhaps people really do believe in evil twin syndrome as it seems that everyone loves to stereotype twins. A gentle explanation that, like all children, yours have good and bad moments, may be required. Or point to them both.

9 **Which one's your favourite?** Honestly, people ask this.

10 **Can you tell them apart?** Yes, because they are my children. And one has curly hair while the other's is straight. Oh, and one's a boy and the other's a girl.

❝ It's like celebrity *Groundhog Day*. Everybody just says exactly the same thing. ❞

Rob, dad to Oscar and Ivy, 21 months

❝ We tend to add about an hour when we go out shopping because we get stopped by that many people. I love it, and today the boys actually smiled at a lady and it was really lovely. Even at work (my partner is on maternity leave) I'm finding I'm getting in late because so many people are stopping me in the corridor to ask about the boys! ❞

Jenny, mum to Ollie and Elliott, ten weeks; Vincent, 22; Christopher, 25; and Elizabeth, 28

66 I've had more than one person peer into the buggy and say, 'That one's bigger than that one. How can they be twins?' Another person told me I needed a dog. 99

Jo, mum to Isla and Sassi, four; and Shea, six

66 People are fascinated by twins. After waiting so long for ours I felt it was a sweet irony that every single day someone would stop me and tell me how beautiful my children are. I never minded. 99

Jayne, mum to Thomas and Holly, 11 months

66 When they were really tiny I had them in a pram top-to-toe (they looked like the Jack in a pack of cards) and people would see one, go to say 'ahh!', and then see the other. Sometimes they would go a bit crazy in astonishment that there was another in there (or cry). I had an amazing moment when the twins were about one and my older boy was having a full-on looney lying-down fit on the street in a busy market. A very well-dressed businessman in his fifties came over, tapped me on the shoulder and told me that it would be all right, and that he had grown-up twin boys and an older boy, too. It was very sweet and entirely unexpected. 99

Jessica, mum to Nat and Joss, four; and Teddy, six

66 When the girls were tiny they got so much attention that my son insisted on going out in fancy dress. Finally, everyone noticed him. 99

Steve, dad to Hannah and Eve, two; and Fergus, four

66 I tended to find that people made negative comments when they stopped me in the street with the buggy such as 'I don't

know how you cope', and I always tried to reply positively because I didn't want my son Ben to have the perception that it was all a big struggle. When people asked about the girls I'd get Ben to tell them their names or remember how old they were and say how lucky they were to have a big brother. "

Emma, mum to Amelie and Jessica, 23 months;
and Ben, three

Being out and about with your babies can leave you basking on a parental pedestal or restraining your inner Rottweiler. Whatever your mood, you'll never be lonely.

Chapter 16

Twin Health and Development

For every parent of twins, the first year brings a barrage of life-changing experiences, heightened emotions and a whole host of issues that it had never previously crossed your mind to worry about. Hopefully, as every month passes, life will start to feel a little easier and more manageable, and as your twins' first year progresses you will also start to focus less on how much sleep you're all getting and more on their development. Watching your little ones learning to smile, babble, become mobile and grapple with solid foods is a wonderful time, and parents can feel justifiably proud at the incredible strides their children take in their first year.

But a graph of life for any of us rarely runs in a straight line, and for every milestone celebrated, there is likely to be parental uncertainty about what is 'normal' and what your children 'should' be doing at this stage. The fact that you have two babies to compare with each other can complicate matters.

Most families experience the setback of illness at some point, especially during the winter months, and this can impact on routines, feeding and overall development for a while. Parents of twins have the unique joy of either having two babies ill at the same time or 'illness relay', where just as one twin shakes off a cold or cough, the other one gets it and the whole process starts again.

This chapter cannot hope to cover all the blips in that graph, but offers a few tips for dealing with some of the more common developmental and health issues that your twins may face in their first year. There are also a few things to watch out for to ward off more serious health problems.

Common health problems

As with all health advice, please be aware that this is general information and is not intended to be a substitute for the opinion of a qualified health professional. Always follow your instincts and if you are concerned about your babies' health, see your GP or call an ambulance.

Fever

Having a hot and unhappy baby – or two – is extremely worrying and it is often difficult to know when you should seek medical help.

You will probably know when your babies have a temperature – they are likely to be hot to the touch and out of sorts. Use a digital thermometer to check your instincts. This is placed in your baby's armpit for about 15 seconds and should give you an accurate temperature, but make sure you follow the instructions carefully.

A fever is considered 37.5°C or more and is a sign of an infection or other illness. If your child's temperature is only slightly above normal (a normal temperature is about 36.4°C) and they don't have any other symptoms, you can help to make them more comfortable.

Make sure they get plenty of drinks to avoid dehydration. If you're breastfeeding, then breast milk is best.

You should contact your GP if:

▶ Your child has other signs of illness in addition to a raised temperature

▶ Your baby's temperature is 38°C or higher if they're under three months, or 39°C or higher if they're three to 12 months

Your GP may suggest using liquid infant paracetamol or ibuprofen to bring down a temperature. Make sure you give the correct dosage for your babies' ages; this will be printed on the packaging. You should check your baby's temperature half an hour after giving the medicine and then monitor it every two to three hours.

Coughs and colds

Coughs and colds are an almost unavoidable problem and, although these are usually relatively short term and minor, they can be very upsetting for your babies and exhausting to deal with as a parent. If your babies develop symptoms at the same time, it can be difficult to soothe and comfort them both or one may pass it to the other, so no sooner does one baby recover than the other baby develops exactly the same symptoms and off you go again, with disrupted sleep and the worry of having an unwell baby.

Premature babies can find it particularly difficult to fight off coughs and colds because their immune system and lungs did not have time to fully mature before they were born.

Precautions to minimise the risks of developing colds and to avoid colds worsening into more serious conditions:

▶ Wash your hands frequently and make sure other siblings do the same

▶ Keep surfaces clean

▶ Regularly wash the babies' toys to avoid infection

▶ Ask friends or relatives with colds to stay away until they have recovered

▶ Avoid smoking anywhere near your babies or their environment

▶ Catch sneezes and coughs in a tissue

Bronchiolitis

Bronchiolitis is the inflammation of the small airways in the lungs that leads to a build up of mucus and causes breathing difficulties. It can often begin with cold-like symptoms and is a common infection that affects babies and young children, often caused by a respiratory syncytial virus infection.

Premature babies or those born with lung or heart problems are particularly at risk and might need extra care if they develop bronchiolitis.

The Twins and Multiple Birth Association has produced the following guide to help parents spot key symptoms and seek early medical help:

▶ **F** – Fast breathing or shallow breathing. Your babies may also look as if they are working harder to breathe by sucking in the area under their ribs or there might be a slight pause between breaths

▶ **A** – Appetite loss or problems with feeding

▶ **C** – Cough, particularly a rasping cough

▶ **T** – Temperature, often a higher temperature than you would expect with a cold. Anything over 38.5°C

If your babies are having problems breathing, seek medical help immediately. Bronchiolitis can often be fairly mild and is usually treated at home, but if there are breathing problems it may be necessary to treat the baby – or babies – in hospital.

> ❝ When the boys were four weeks old they had a tickly cough and on/off laboured breathing, which had gone on for a few days and just seemed to keep on going. Arthur seemed more affected and was very pale, so we were going to take them to the doctor the following day. However, that evening Arthur went very still and white as a sheet, and didn't seem to be breathing – he was, as it turned out but it was just very shallow – so we rang an ambulance and he was taken into hospital. Thomas was also admitted and both were put into oxygen tents on the bed (very scary) and then admitted to the intensive care unit. Arthur had a part-collapsed lung. They were in the intensive care unit for five or six days. It was a very stressful time and quite a shock as it's not really a condition that you're made aware of ahead of time. One thing the doctors did say was that it was late to get it as most cases are in the autumn or winter, but this was spring, so it can happen any time. ❞

Peter, dad to Thomas and Arthur, 18 months;
and Edward, three

Teething

Most babies begin teething at around six months, but, as with all milestones, this varies considerably, and teeth can first start coming through from four months or can take as long as 12 months. The bottom front teeth are the first to appear, followed by the top front teeth. While this is an exciting time, it can also throw a spanner in the works in terms of sleep and routine, as new teeth often cause your babies discomfort and pain, and can result in a lot of grizzling. It also adds a new hazard to breastfeeding.

Teething rings, especially ones that can be cooled in the fridge first, can give your babies some comfort. Also, teething gels that can be rubbed directly on to the gums can help numb the pain. Always check you have a gel designed specifically for young children and ask your pharmacist to advise you. A small dose of liquid paracetamol or ibuprofen, specifically designed for children, may also help. Make sure you follow the dosage instructions that come with the medicine. If in doubt, check with your GP or pharmacist.

Bacterial meningitis

This is not a common problem but it is extremely serious and it is essential for all parents to know the symptoms so that you can get medical help quickly if necessary. Any case of suspected meningitis should be treated as an emergency.

Meningitis (either bacterial or viral) is the infection and inflammation of the protective membranes (meninges) that surround the brain and spinal cord, which in some cases can damage the nerves and brain.

Common symptoms of meningitis in babies:

- ▶ A high fever, with cold hands and feet
- ▶ Vomiting and a refusal to feed
- ▶ Agitation and not wanting to be picked up
- ▶ Being drowsy, floppy and unresponsive
- ▶ Grunting or breathing rapidly
- ▶ An unusual high-pitched or moaning cry
- ▶ Pale, blotchy skin and a red rash that doesn't fade when a glass is rolled over it
- ▶ A tense, bulging soft spot on their head (a fontanelle)
- ▶ A stiff neck and a dislike of bright lights
- ▶ Convulsions or seizures

This condition can come on very suddenly and your baby may not necessarily display all the symptoms. Don't wait for certain better-known signs, such as a rash, to appear. If your baby is unwell and getting worse, call an ambulance.

Flat head syndrome

This condition, also known as plagiocephaly, occurs when one side of a baby's head is flattened and therefore looks asymmetrical. Babies' skulls are still soft enough to be moulded and can change shape if there is constant pressure, such as from the same sleeping position. Once the head shape flattens, the baby will favour that side as it is more comfortable, which can make the problem worse.

Flat head syndrome is more prevalent in twins, possibly because prematurity and lying for extended periods of time in a neonatal unit are more likely. In the busy weeks following the babies' arrival at home, it can be surprisingly easy to miss the fact that occasionally both, but usually one, of your babies has got a misshapen head. Although very worrying for parents, it is a condition that, with some help, will usually correct itself.

Steps to try at home to counteract flat head syndrome:

▶ Tummy time. Young babies don't always enjoy being put on their tummies, as initially they don't have the strength to hold their heads up. You can support their chests to make them more comfortable, or lay them on top of you.

▶ Change the position of cot toys or mobiles to encourage your babies to turn their heads in the other direction.

▶ Put a toy or distraction on the changing mat to encourage your babies to turn away from the flattened side.

▶ During the day, put your baby in a sling or a sloping chair to encourage them to look in different directions and to keep the pressure off the flattened side.

▶ When you are feeding, make sure that your babies have to turn away from their flattened side to take the bottle or breast.

▶ Remember that, for safety reasons, your babies should still be put down to sleep on their backs.

If your baby is having difficulty moving its head to the other side, then your doctor is likely to recommend seeing a physiotherapist.

The other option, not generally available on the NHS, is for your baby to wear a specially made corrective helmet, which can be considered from about five months if progress has not been made using the techniques above. These helmets have to be worn almost constantly to be effective and opinion is divided about whether the head will correct itself over time anyway without the need for one. However, many parents feel they have worked miracles on their babies and highly recommend them.

Bonding with your twins

Parents tend to assume that they will fall hopelessly in love with their babies the moment they set eyes on them – and many do. But it is quite normal for that special mummy– or daddy–baby bond to take longer to form.

With two babies to care for, parents of twins often do not have the luxury of spending hours staring into their babies' eyes and holding them, because there's always another baby waiting for the same treatment. Added to which, one or both babies may be in special care, and worry and stress may overshadow bonding. You are likely to feel very protective about your tiny babies, which is a form of bonding in itself, but many parents of premature twins find it takes a bit longer for the gushy, all-encompassing love to hit them.

A bonding complication that is unique to parents of twins is that you may not feel the same way about both babies. Sometimes parents get in the habit of looking after a baby each and, without being conscious of doing so, build up a stronger relationship with one twin. If one baby is more demanding or cries a lot, you may start to resent it and favour the 'easier' twin.

> ❝ It is not uncommon for a mother not to immediately bond with her babies. We are all led to believe that we have to instantly fall in love with our babies and if it doesn't happen it feels as if you've failed to achieve what should be a basic human instinct. However, these things can take time and the attachment and bonding does form over the coming days and weeks. You need to remind yourself that you are extra tired and run down – feelings that can take precedence over initial bonding. With twins, you have 50 per cent less time with your babies and you may feel that the practical duties are crowding out just spending time with a baby on your lap. If you have picked up one baby, you may feel guilty that you aren't picking up the other one, and resent the fact that your time feels so rationed. ❞
>
> *Dr Saima Latif, chartered psychologist, and mum to Haris and Faris, seven*

Don't panic if you don't feel the way you expected to when your babies are born. Concentrate on caring for them and spending as much time as you can with each baby, and slowly the bonds should form. There's no magic formula to this except to enjoy your babies and wait for the feelings to come. If you become aware that you are bonding more with one baby than the other, make sure you change your routine so that you spend more time with the second baby in order to get to know each other and build up your relationship.

> 66 At our 20-week scan we discovered Twin 2 (John) had a cleft palate. As a result, most of the attention was on him – family would ask about Twin 2 and, I realise now, that Twin 1 (Elizabeth) was hardly spoken about because she was always OK. Ironically when they were born Elizabeth had stopped growing about two weeks beforehand and was smaller than John.
>
> It was really hard. I didn't bother breastfeeding John because I knew I wouldn't be able to feed him, but I really wanted to breastfeed Elizabeth, and I struggled and so did she. It was a very negative experience and I remember lots of tears. It has taken 18 months for me to really love her and I say that with a heavy heart. We put so much energy into worrying about John that Elizabeth was left out. 99
>
> *Sara, mum to John and Elizabeth, two.*

In some cases, the lack of bonding you may be feeling could be an indictor of postnatal depression. If you are feeling low, withdrawn and are not getting any pleasure from your babies, see your GP. (For more information about postnatal depression, see Chapter 14.)

Communication

It is well known that twins are sometimes slower to develop language skills than single children, and on average toddler twins will be about six months behind their peers. Many of the reasons behind this are obvious: parents find it harder to give one-to-one eye contact with two babies and tend to talk to both of them at the same time (or look at one baby while talking to the other), twins spend much of their time together so it is natural for them to copy each other's babble rather than their parents' more mature speech, and there is simply less undivided attention for each child.

Bear in mind that lots of twins suffer no delay at all in their ability to communicate and don't forget that all milestone guides are approximate – you shouldn't worry too much if your babies aren't doing exactly what other babies are doing. There are plenty of things you can do during their first year to encourage your twins' speech development. The first year is about making as much individual eye contact and spending as much direct talking time as you can with each baby.

Ideas from the National Literacy Trust on your babies' communication milestones in the first year and how to encourage their speech:

▶ **By three months** – Your babies already recognise the sound of their mother's voice before they are born and are aware of language within days of their birth. Babies are fascinated by faces and will copy movements, such as sticking out your tongue. Make sure you look directly at one baby when you talk to them – it's never too soon to chat and sing together. Always respond when one or both of your babies is trying to communicate. At this stage your babies may watch your face while you talk, turn towards your voice and sometimes join in and start making cooing and gurgling noises.

▶ **By six months** – Your babies will start to make noises and will be keen to engage with adults talking, singing or reading books without noise in the background. Listen to your babies' babbles and respond. Leave time to let them respond to what you say. Take it in turns to 'have a chat', perhaps while you are changing one of the babies' nappies so you can make good eye contact in a quiet environment. Once you start weaning, use feeding as a time to get short bursts of eye contact and have a chat.

▶ **By one year** – Your babies will have found other ways to communicate now, perhaps by waving and pointing as well as making sounds. They may be starting to understand routines and simple words and activities. Try action rhymes, such as 'wind the bobbin up' or 'pat-a-cake'. Each baby may now look at you when you call their name and they may be learning how to get your attention by shouting, pointing or making other noises if they can't reach something. When reading, give each baby a book and let them show you what interests them.

Milestones

Your twins are two different people, but it is often assumed by others, or even parents themselves, that they will develop at the same rate. There can be big gaps between one twin crawling, walking or getting their first tooth and the second twin doing the same thing. As a parent it can be worrying to see one baby happily bum-shuffling around the room while the other one is still static, but their progress will almost always even out or the twin who has been developing more slowly in one area may be more advanced in another. It is really hard to avoid comparisons when you have children of the same age, but be careful of labelling one baby as being 'ahead' or 'behind' the other. Encourage each baby at whatever stage they have reached.

It is not unusual for your twins to be rather different sizes. Some twins' weights vary dramatically at birth; others are born a similar weight but one grows and develops quicker than the other.

> 66 Harri weighed 50 per cent more than Gethin and there was a constant lag in their development. Gethin was usually a month or two behind Harri on everything until it came to linguistic development and then he was the one ahead. It extended to everything. Gethin would just catch up with Harri in the amount of milk he was drinking and I'd get them on the same routine, and then Harri's demands would change and he'd be on different sized bottles again – they never quite became parallel. 99
>
> *Meryl, mum to Harri and Gethin, seven*

> 66 At 11 months Tommy is now almost walking and weighs 20 lb, while Lizzie is making no attempt to crawl and weighs 15 lb, so now I get asked what the age gap is and all I can say is 'one minute'. I heard someone the other day at a play session exclaim, 'Oh look at those two, they could almost be brother and sister.' 99
>
> *Linda, mum to Tommy and Lizzie, 11 months*

Sometimes, parental instinct or the comments of a friend or health visitor may alert you to the fact that something is not quite right, in which case do not hesitate to approach your GP with your concerns. New parents can be worried that they will be considered fussy or over-protective, but you know your children better than anyone and if you feel something is wrong, trust your instincts and do all you can to persuade someone to listen to you.

66 Ivy struggled with balance, and had glue ear and adenoids, which made her breathing at night difficult. We knew right from the moment she was born that something wasn't right, but no one would take us seriously. Because the twins were our first, we'd get condescending comments about being first-time parents and were made to feel that we didn't know anything. We saw over 20 doctors and finally we had a chance meeting at our twins club with an ear, nose and throat specialist, who listened to us. A few weeks ago Ivy had an operation and has been a different child ever since. It was really hard to see her struggling while her twin, Oscar, taught himself to crawl and walk. You could see Ivy looking at him thinking 'I want to do that'. Now, at last, she can start to catch up. 99

Rob, dad to Ivy and Oscar, 21 months

66 I don't want anyone to be paranoid about it, but if you feel that your child is constantly missing milestones and that something isn't right, it is worth questioning.

I wish that I had followed my instincts a bit and had made a fuss. If someone had told me my twins would be autistic I would have been terrified, but actually day to day the boys are lovely, we have a lot of fun with them and they are very rewarding. You have to accept that life is a bit different. In the end, the child that you imagine you will have is not the one that you will always get, but you will love them anyway. 99

Alex, mum to James and Harry, four

Parents of premature twins know that their babies are likely to be late in hitting their milestones and may have additional concerns that prematurity has affected their children's development in a more fundamental way – something that should be closely monitored by health professionals. When working out how your twins are progressing, they will use an 'adjusted' birth date – that of their due date, not the actual day they were born – to take into account their prematurity. It is hard not to compare your babies with other children of the same age, but your twins have a lot of catching up to do. Measure them by their own progress – which is often amazing! Hopefully by the age of two, premature babies will have caught up and can revert to their birth date, although in very premature babies this catch-up date can be extended to the age of three.

> 66 They are really diddy. When we got to eight months you expect them to be rolling about, but they were still like four or five month olds – which in a way they were. Henley wouldn't weight-bear on his legs, but he was the first to take steps at 14 months. They are quite intelligent, but you can't just forget about those three months at the beginning. At playgroup last week a mother was telling her daughter to be careful of the 'babies' – it turned out she was five months younger than my 'babies'! 99
>
> *Clare, mum to Henley and Riley, 19 months, born at 29 weeks + four days; Lexi, three; and Kaysie, nine*

Yikes!

No other profession takes you as deeply into a world of worry, fretting and self-doubt than that of parenthood. There are so many things that *could* happen that at times it can feel a bit overwhelming. This is where being a parent of twins becomes a massive advantage, because for the most part, you just don't have time to think about it. Life for at least the first few months is all about getting through the sleep deprivation, making sure everyone is fed and clothed, and ensuring that someone in the house is functional enough to earn a living.

> 66 I'd be running round like an idiot for 16 or 17 hours a day. You almost don't notice that it's getting easier. It is a gradual thing – you realise that the twins are three months old and that you're all ok. Then four months gets a bit easier, and five months a bit easier than that, but you don't have the time to stand back and ask 'Are we all right, can we do anything differently', you just have to get on with it and keep going. 99
>
> *James, dad to Rosie and Elliott, seven months; and Robin, three*

So if you've been able to read this chapter and are feeling worried by a whole host of new things to consider, give yourself a big pat on the back. Not only is your head far enough above water to take all this in, but you have time to think about it. Hooray! Life with your twins must be getting easier.

Chapter 17

Weaning

At last! This is the really fun part. Not only do you get to combine all sorts of unlikely flavours and textures in the name of nutrition, but you will also find out how they look on your wall.

Babies are surprisingly open to new flavours, once they've got over the shock that there is more to life than warm milk. You will have endless comic moments watching their expressions as alien flavours meet their taste buds, so keep the camera handy. Now you have a whole new set of likes and dislikes to keep track of, which you can guarantee will rarely overlap. Do keep trying with foods that have been rejected though, as they might get the seal of approval a few days later.

When to start?

Most babies are ready to wean at six months, but will continue to get most of their nutrition from milk until they are about 12 months. Initially, food will be used largely as decoration or face paint, but the odd mouthful will find its way to the right place and your babies (and maybe even you) will have quite a lot of fun getting used to this exciting new world of food.

Signs that your babies are probably ready to be weaned:

▶ They can sit up by themselves and keep their heads steady

▶ They swallow their food – you'll soon know if they can't because they'll push it all out again with their tongues

▶ They have enough coordination to grab what food they want and put it in their mouths

Babies will often watch intently as you eat your food and may try to grab it for themselves; this can be another sign that they are ready or it may be general curiosity. If you think your babies are ready to be weaned before six months, discuss this with your health visitor first.

Getting started

If there is a history of allergies in your family, you should consult your GP before starting the weaning process. Never leave your babies unattended while they are eating.

There are two general approaches to weaning, although it's increasingly common to use a mixture of both methods. You have the option of feeding your babies purees and mashed-up food with a spoon, or you can adopt baby-led weaning – a slightly grandiose term for letting your babies feed themselves. For parents of twins, there are pros and cons to both approaches.

Baby-led weaning is less labour intensive in terms of preparing and pureeing food, but some parents worry that they can't keep track of how much their babies have eaten very easily (or think they've done brilliantly and then find it all squished behind the high chair seat later) and are concerned that they wouldn't be able to cope if both babies choked on pieces of broccoli at the same time. However, if your babies take to baby-led weaning you will have your hands free to eat lunch yourself, which is quite useful.

Feeding your babies pureed food has the advantage that you are putting food straight into your babies' mouths (even if it sometimes comes straight back out again, or meets firmly pursed lips) and is a little less messy. However, you will spend quite a bit more time preparing food, if you choose to home cook it.

> 66 Weaning is now referred to as complementary feeding, as in the first year babies get most of their nutrition from their milk. Appetites vary massively day to day and the important thing is to try to stay relaxed about weaning as it's easy to get stressed about it.
>
> There is absolutely no evidence that baby-led weaning is better and no evidence to say that there's anything wrong with it, either. To use the best of both approaches can work best for your babies – that's certainly what I did with mine. 99
>
> **Dr Frankie Phillips, dietician with special interest in children's nutrition, and mum to Natalie and Sian, seven**

Weaning two babies simultaneously is very messy, so be prepared.

Tips to (slightly) reduce the chaos of weaning:

▶ The more elaborate your high chairs are, the more there is to clean. Many parents recommend basic, plastic high chairs for ease of cleaning. Avoid anything with lots of crevices or fabric.

▶ Stand the highchairs on an old, washable shower curtain or a large piece of plastic to catch the debris.

▶ Invest in some long-sleeved bibs. Some parents also put a pelican bib (cleanable in a dishwasher) over the top of the long-sleeved bib.

▶ Save really messy or smelly (i.e. fish) meals for just before bath time.

▶ Remove a few layers of clothes at feeding time. Try feeding the babies in their vests or nappies or naked. OK, the latter may not actually reduce the mess.

▶ Get a dog.

▶ Don't stress about it. Everyone has their own 'mess threshold', but does it really matter if your babies have to wear a top with the odd spaghetti Bolognese stain on it for a few hours? If the answer is yes, then accept you are going to be doing considerably more laundry for a while.

The first day of 'solids' can be a slight anti-climax. For a start, the food is not solid. Secondly, the quantities involved are tiny. For the first week or so, you will be giving the babies very simple foods, such as pureed bananas, cooked apples, pears, carrots or sweet potatoes (see page 239). They are likely to want only a teaspoon or so as they get used to the different tastes and textures of their food.

You will continue to give them their normal milk intake throughout most of the weaning process, although if they are eating well, demand for milk may naturally fall. Remember that most of their nutrition will come from their milk until they are about 12 months, so try not to worry about how much solid food they are consuming, especially in the early stages. You should take your cue from your babies. When they are ready for more, they will ask for it. You are choosing what your babies have to eat, but they will tell you how much they want.

Start with one solid meal a day for the first few weeks, then move up to two solid meals a day and, as your babies' appetites demand it, three.

You can use cow's milk in recipes, but it must not be used as a main drink for your babies until they are 12 months old. They should continue with regular feeds of either breast milk or formula. You can give them water in a cup with a lid and spout to have with their food from six months.

‶ I started weaning with purees (one bowl, one spoon) but Alex hated it once he realised he could do it himself, so after about two weeks we went to baby-led weaning and it has been brilliant for us. I have a big shower curtain that I put on the floor and that I can wash in the washing machine as it is very messy, but really they took to it brilliantly and it was great as we could all eat together and I finally got to drink hot tea! ″

Lindsay, mum to Serafina and Alex, 22 months

‶ I started off with different water cups, spoons, everything, but halfway through feeding I'd get confused about who had which spoon and I'm sure I muddled them up anyway. A few weeks ago I thought forget it, and now I just use one. ″

Katie, mum to Keira and Gracie, 11 months; and Layla, five

‶ I started trying to do way too much food and after a projectile vom session after a mix of carrot, banana, yoghurt and broccoli, I thought I needed to give us all a break. I went back to just giving them some baby porridge (easier as it's just mixed with water not formula or breast milk) in the mornings and mixing in some pureed fruit if I have some or a mashed banana.

We have built up gradually and they are having two sessions a day now with veg or fruit. I get mangos from the market, which are cheap and overripe and perfect for just pureeing up and freezing, plus things like frozen peas which don't need any prep.

I feel that baby-led weaning is a bit of a pretentious phrase for giving them bits of lovingly steamed butternut squash to throw on the floor. I'm also nervous doing that as I can't watch both of them like a hawk at all times in case they choke. A slice of toast and a bit of banana is as far as it's got now and I'm comfortable with that. ″

Gabby, mum to Astrid and Florrie, seven months

First foods

Once you've got through the first few weeks, there are loads of things you can try your babies on. Build up gradually, but don't be afraid to try new flavours and don't feel you have to mask tricky flavours with sweet ones. Even unexpected stuff like lemons can prove acceptable and they might love broccoli all by itself, who knows? Don't panic if it seems like nothing is being eaten because they are still getting all the nutrition they need from their usual milk rations.

Don't add sugar or salt to your babies' food and avoid stock cubes, which are very salty. Babies' kidneys can only process small amounts of salt a day (less than 1 g a day for babies under seven months).

Nut butters or ground nuts are fine from six months, but whole nuts should be avoided as they are a choking hazard. If you are concerned about a potential allergic reaction, talk to your GP or health visitor before experimenting with that particular food.

You will quickly build up confidence in what you are prepared to try your babies on, but here are a few suggestions to start you off.

Suggestions for first foods:

▶ Banana

▶ Avocado

▶ Soft, cooked vegetables, such as carrot or sweet potato

▶ Cooked apple or pear

▶ Baby rice or cereal mixed with breast milk or formula

▶ Cut-up cucumber

Suggestions for foods to move on to:

► Grated raw vegetables

► Mashed-up hard-boiled egg

► Cheese slices

► Peeled and sliced fruit such as melon and strawberries, or quartered grapes

► Cooked pasta

► Mashed-up fish (check for bones)

► Toast or bread soldiers

► Soft, cooked meat, such as chicken

► Dry cereal

► Halved cherry tomatoes

► Breadsticks

❝ This period offers a precious window, which lasts from about six months to ten months where your babies are open to new tastes and textures. Try to move quickly through textures. Research shows that babies who are exposed to and accept lumpy food early on do end up with a better diet when they are older. Also, if your babies spit out food one day, don't assume they won't ever like it. Try it again a few days later and keep trying. ❞

Dr Frankie Phillips, dietician with special interest in children's nutrition, and mum to Natalie and Sian, seven

> 66 Mine ate anything I stuck in their mouths pretty much, so I felt confident about introducing lots of flavours. You can also add a pinch of turmeric, cinnamon, fresh basil, etc. to batches for more interest. My boys especially loved sweet potato, carrots, swede, parsnips, mango, pear and apple. Tinned tuna is great for mixing with veg. Mine even loved Brussels sprouts! Other fish I used was frozen boneless cod steaks and haddock. You can just get one or two out whilst batch cooking to mix in.
>
> I didn't bother freezing tiny portions of things into cube trays, I just used small plastic pots, which are ten a penny in supermarkets. Make up dinners and freeze in a portion for two. It will save you time mixing things together and you just defrost one pot for dinner (or two as they get older). As long as you make sure you give them enough dairy, protein and veg, etc. you can use dinners in rotation. 99
>
> *Kaz, mum to Reuben and Nathaniel, five*

Parents understandably worry that their babies are going to choke on their food, and there is a fair amount of coughing and spluttering involved in weaning, as well as the odd vomiting protest. However, babies have been cleverly designed with their gag reflex further forwards in their mouths than adults and if food gets too far back it will be coughed up pronto. Make sure you always watch your babies when they are eating, just in case, and never leave them unattended.

Calm down, dear

There's something about the weaning process that brings out the Italian mama in us. Faced with the responsibility of introducing their twins to the world of food, some mummies go slightly mad, cooking feasts that bring together flavours from across the globe, leaving no culinary stone unturned, often at the expense of resting or enjoying their babies. Partners come home to find the fridge full of tempting grub, only to be told to keep their hands off because it's all for the twins. Supper is leftovers from lunch – which is possibly still on the floor.

Mummies can get a little competitive over whose homemade organic meal is the *most* homemade. You mean you didn't make your own stock and whip up that custard from scratch? Tsk, tsk. Things can get a little out of hand in the rush to answer nature's most basic call: to nourish our little ones.

Try to resist. Give yourself a break and don't compare your efforts with anyone else's, especially mums of single babies. If you can manage to cook up some homemade food, or adapt what you are eating for the babies, then brilliant. If not, there are plenty of good, organic (if you feel the need), unsalted, ready-made baby foods out there, which will do your twins no end of good, too. Not to mention all those finger foods that can be whipped up in no time at all without even having to look at a cooker.

‟ When we started weaning, I tried to be supermum. All I could think about was making perfect home-cooked food for the babies and I'd spend all their naptimes making food. The list of ingredients they had in their first week of weaning was ridiculous! The high I would get from them eating my food was just incredible, but then there was the absolute low when they wouldn't even try it and threw it on the floor. I was completely exhausted and realised that I'd got quite low, which was not like me at all. I talked to other friends and realised that I needed to relax more and not worry about being perfect. When I did that the twins were still happy and healthy, and absolutely as they should be. I didn't want to waste time feeling low and miss these wonderful months with my children. 〟

Lucie, mum to Ivy and Oscar, 21 months

It is an unwritten rule of parenting that the more effort you put into food, the less likely it is to be eaten. Have fun with this window of culinary experimentation while it lasts, but keep the cordon bleu for yourselves once in a while – your partner won't believe how good food tastes from a plate.

Chapter 18

Safely on the Move

You are now entering a phase when the only place to put a cup of tea in your sitting room is on a shelf approximately 3 cm from the ceiling. Complicated cupboard locks have turned your kitchen into a Bank of England vault and you have to allow an extra ten minutes to get to the toilet in order to undo a maze of safety gates along the way.

In the course of this year, your twins will go from being rather puny and immobile newborns to rolling, sitting, grasping and possibly even walking little people. And, of course, while one is putting the dog's plastic bone in her mouth, the other is crawling over to investigate exactly how the television works, using the flex as a useful handhold to get to the screen.

Your trips out are probably far more active now, with the babies keen to be liberated from the pushchair and to explore exciting things like playgrounds, cafes, toilets and rubbish bins.

Making your home a safe place to explore and rethinking how to manage your activities when you are out and about are essential to help you maintain your peace of mind while allowing your twins to indulge their natural curiosity.

Twin-proofing your home

When viewed through health-and-safety goggles, most homes would probably fail even the most preliminary of inspections. Once you are aware of the safety pitfalls, it is easy to become a little paranoid about the array of accidents that can be triggered by a momentary lack of supervision. Happily, simply being aware of potential hazards goes a long way towards preventing them, so try to keep the risks in perspective.

The most important first step for parents of twins is to have somewhere safe that you can put your babies if you need to go to the toilet, make a drink, answer the phone or take a couple of minutes' out. This can be done fairly easily by putting the babies in their cots or by creating a playpen or by using a travel cot in a downstairs room.

"I'd recommend the double playpen. It's a lifesaver with multiple toddlers. You get two hexagonal playpens, and join them together to form a shape to fit your room. If square, it's 6 x 6 feet. It's so big that we can keep almost all of their toys in there, so it's more like a playroom than a prison. We use it after meals so we can clear the mess up without it spreading further; during cooking when they'd prefer to be under your feet or destroying your kitchen; and generally when it all gets too much. We keep it open most of the time. It's been up since they've been mobile. They are still generally happy to be inside it, and haven't yet climbed out. I don't know how we'll cope when they do. "

Nicola, mum to Jonathan and Abigail, 20 months

"I had a travel cot downstairs when they started crawling and I filled it with those plastic balls you get at soft play, so I could put them in there for a bit. What we basically did though was baby proof our house and give them pretty much free rein of it. For cooking I put them in their high chairs with spoons and things to bang, but otherwise if I needed the loo or something I just left them in the living room. Now, of course, they want to come with me and supervise! "

Lindsay, mum to Serafina and Alex, 22 months

It's Twins! Now What?

It is not possible to eliminate all risks from our everyday lives, nor would most people want to, but you can minimise the chances of a serious injury by spending a little bit of time assessing your home and making a few small changes to improve its safety.

Falls

Every day, 45 toddlers are taken to hospital because they've had a serious fall. These can happen anywhere – from tripping over on a flat surface to tumbling off a sofa or from a window or from heavy objects falling on your child.

Some tips for preventing falls:

▶ Do not leave a baby unattended on any raised surface – even if you think they can't roll off. There's always a first time.

▶ Don't put a bouncing cradle or similar on a table or worktop as they could bounce off the edge.

▶ Fit safety stair gates and attach safety catches to upstairs windows (which restrict the opening to 6.5 centimetres), but make sure they can be opened fully in an emergency. Do not put anything under a window that can be climbed on.

▶ Attach heavy objects such as book shelves and media units to the wall so they can't be pulled over onto your babies.

▶ Do not leave anything on the stairs that my be tripped over. Check there is no room for a small child to crawl through any banisters.

Scalds and burns

Hot drinks are responsible for the most scalds and burns to young children. About six toddlers are admitted to hospital every day

246

as a result of bad burns. Injury can also be caused by hot bath water, heated appliances, such as hair straighteners, open fires, cigarettes and matches and many other hot surfaces. Babies have much more delicate skin than adults so extra care must be taken to protect them.

Safeguarding tips to prevent scalds and burns:

▶ Keep hot drinks away from your babies. It may feel like you are constantly drinking luke warm tea, but a hot drink can still burn a baby 15 minutes after it has been made.

▶ Take extra care at bathtime. Don't leave a young child alone in the bathroom. When running a bath, fill with cold water first and test the temperature with your elbow. It should feel warm, not hot or cold.

▶ Use rear hotplates on your hob and turn panhandles away from the front of the cooker. Use a cordless kettle or one with a short or curly flex pushed to the back of the worktop.

▶ Keep small children out of the kitchen whenever possible.

▶ Keep curling tongs, irons and hair straighteners out of reach when they are in use and cooling down.

▶ Keep matches, cigarette lighters and candles out of sight and reach of children.

Fire

Breathing in poisonous smoke is much more likely to cause a fatality than being burnt by the fire itself, so setting up an escape plan and making sure you have smoke alarms which work in your home are important first steps in protecting your family.

Tips to prevent a fire:

▸ Install a working smoke alarm on every level of your house. Check the batteries each week. Never remove the batteries. Some Fire and Rescue Services will install smoke alarms free of charge.

▸ Have an established safety routine at night. Close doors and windows, switch off appliances and put out any cigarettes or candles.

Poisoning

Most poisoning accidents involve medicines, household products (such as cleaning fluids) and cosmetics.

Tips to prevent poisoning:

▸ Fit carbon monoxide wherever there is a flame-burning appliance (such as a gas boiler) or an open fire. Make sure your appliances are services regularly.

▸ Bear in mind that children can be better at opening "child resistant" containers than adults. Keep medication and household chemicals, including cleaning products, out of sight and reach or locked away safely. Store chemicals in their original containers.

Suffocating and choking

Children can swallow, inhale or choke on items such as small toys, button batteries, peanuts, plastic bags and marbles.

Tips to prevent suffocating and choking:

- Keep small items away from children under three. If you have older children, make sure their toys are kept separately, well away from areas accessed by the babies.

- Keep nappy sacks out of reach and never store them in or around the cot area. They are easy to grasp and can be breathed in by young babies without parents realising.

- Button batteries, such as those used in watches or some toys, pose not only a risk of choking, but if swallowed can kill a young child in a matter of hours. Seek urgent medical help if this happens.

- Keep your babies' cots away from blind cords, which should be kept short and out of reach. Better still, install cordless blinds. Every year one of two children die as a result of becoming entangled in blind cords.

- Do not hang toys or objects, such as drawstring bags on or near a cot.

Drowning

Your children need constant supervision when in or near water. A child can drown in just a few centimetres of water, and is likely to do so silently so you may not have any warning that something is wrong.

Tips to prevent drowning:

- Never leave babies unattended in the bath, even for a moment

- Fill in garden ponds or fence them off. Check your garden fence is secure so that your children can't fall into a neighbour's pond.

- Empty paddling pools when not in use.

Socket covers

Modern 13-amp power sockets have a shutter mechanism that stops accidental connection to a live wire, so it is no longer necessary to have socket covers. However, it is still important to instil in your children the risks associated with electricity and to store electrical equipment away safely when not in use.

Double trouble

With danger lurking under every cushion cover, you may feel it is pretty miraculous to have made it this far. As you will have already discovered, babies are remarkably resilient and, no matter how careful you are, they will have tumbles, falls and scrapes as a result of their natural curiosity and desire to explore.

Hopefully your twins' antics will be memorable, not because of the resultant trip to A&E, but because two inquisitive little people can add up to some very funny situations – although it may take you a few years to fully appreciate the humour. If you are looking at your innocent-seeming twins and wondering why all this is necessary, here are a few stories about some cheeky twins higher up the food chain which might just persuade you that a containment strategy is well worth employing.

> ❝I left them in the front garden with the gate shut, all ready for nursery, while I got the buggy out of the car. My partner Andrew had left a full tin of masonry paint and a brush on the windowsill (obviously not very well sealed). Within three minutes they had managed to paint each other – coat, shoes and hair. There was a little trail of white footprints across the grass, too. It was everywhere. I had to scrub them and their shoes with a green scourer. ❞
>
> *Tracy, mum to Toren and Mairead, six, Edan, two; and Conall, ten*

66 Jake had reflux and once they were eating solids he would always be a bit sick when he'd got down from his high chair and was crawling around after food, which I'd obviously clean up. One day I was in the kitchen loading the dishwasher, continuously glancing into the living room to check the boys were OK. I saw the boys gathered around a blob of something on the floor, so I came into the room thinking it was clean-up time again. It was, but not what I'd expected. Alex had done the most enormous poo, so enormous that a substantial amount had come out of his nappy and dropped out of his trouser leg on to the floor. Jake had been curiously standing over the dollop. When he looked up he had poo all over his face and was smacking his lips as if savouring this new taste sensation. Nice! 99

Sarah, mum to Alex and Jake, six; and Nell, nine

66 I used to keep the snacks on the top shelf of the cupboard. One day when the boys were about two and a half I came downstairs and heard a lot of giggling coming from the kitchen. They'd pulled in a chair from the dining room and Charlie was on it on tiptoe, reaching for the biscuits, egged on by Ted below who was acting as lookout! 99

Jules, mum to Charlie and Ted, five

66 Here's what my little monkeys did in the space of one morning when they were 22 months:

1. Filled their mouths with their brother's Lego
2. Painted the sofa with Sudocrem
3. Threw decorative stones out of the neighbour's flowerbeds
4. Tried to dismantle a school display of a visiting author's work
5. Emptied water cups and lunch over table / selves / floor. 99

Amanda, mum to Freya and Casper, two; Gabriel, seven; and Felix, ten

Moving on up and out

Trips out with your twins are a lot more fun once they start to get interested in their surroundings, but they also present more of a headache in terms of keeping them under surveillance and out of trouble.

Many parents feel quite daunted at the thought of venturing to playgrounds alone once their babies are able to move about independently, but there are a few things you can do to make it a more manageable experience.

How to contain your twins in the great outdoors:

▶ Invest in all-in-one waterproof overalls. Even if your babies can't walk, you can let them explore an enclosed section of your park or playground without worrying about them getting wet, cold or dirty.

▶ If your twins are intent on moving in different directions and you are worried one baby may crawl under the path of a swing or hurl themselves off a slide, put one baby back into the buggy while you concentrate on the other baby. This won't be popular, but is safer than a clonk on the head. You could try telling them: 'It's Evan's turn now. Next it will be your turn.' Then swap them over after five minutes. If it is snack time, the baby in the buggy could have their snack as compensation.

▶ Consider reins or backpacks with a lead. This gives you peace of mind about their safety and whereabouts, but can lead to other problems. When a baby is learning to walk, they will often keep going until they reach the end of the lead – and then fall over. And then cry.

▶ Try to stick with one of your children. You can then quickly scoop up the nearest baby and run after the other one if necessary. There's nothing worse than being in the middle and trying to work out which one to 'save' first.

► Stick to smaller, manageable playgroups or ones where you know the other mums will help you out, such as your local twins group.

It's easy to say, but try not to get too stressed when you are out and about. If the worst that happens is that your twins eat mud, cover themselves in bark chippings and shuffle off with another child's welly then you've had a good day.

Chapter 19

Parenting Twins

If you were to bundle all your emotions, fears and dreams into a backpack and throw it on to a trampoline, you'd start to get some idea of the feelings involved in being a new parent. With twins, of course, that backpack may need to be twice as big and could bounce twice as high.

Joy, love, pride, anxiety, awe, fatigue and despair all ricochet around the newly parental brain for a while as the reality of your new babies and the responsibilities involved in their care start to take root. Once that heady cocktail calms down, parents can begin to address some of the unique issues that raising twins entails, such as how to encourage your children to be individuals whilst also recognising the importance of the twin relationship.

Your children will always be twins, and that is very special, but they will be so many other things, too. As their parents, one of your jobs is to help them show the outside world that not only do they make a lovely pair, but as individuals they have even more talents to offer.

Early bonding with your twins

One of the most joyous experiences of being a new parent is holding your baby close, staring into its eyes and simply revelling in the fact that you have created this little miracle. But what do you do when you've got another little miracle in a bouncy chair next to you who'd also like to stare lovingly into your eyes?

Grab any time you can to make individual eye contact with your babies – changing nappies is a good time to do this. You can also have a little sing-song and 'chat' while you're at it.

Parents of twins quickly become used to the fact that a lot of happy moments are slightly tinged with guilt, because in focusing on one baby, the other inevitably misses out. Or you sit cross-eyed on the sofa, trying to achieve the impossible of giving two people undivided attention at once. As we heard in Chapter 16, the issue of bonding unexpectedly slowly with your twins can give some parents real heartache and concern.

> " You can feed two at a time, push two children on a swing at the same time, but you can't make eye contact with two babies at the same time and we know that eye contact is really important in the development of social communication abilities. It is entirely possible that one baby will have worked out that eye contact is a good way of getting attention and is more socially engaging than the other baby, and as a parent we need to make sure that each baby receives plenty of eye contact regardless of whether they demand it or not.
>
> It is not just about eye contact with adults. It is important that twins lie with each other. They won't get as much eye contact from adult carers, but they will get it from each other, too. "
>
> *Dr Sarah Helps, consultant clinical psychologist and family therapist, and mum to 12-year-old twins*

What your babies may lack in parental attention, however, they make up for with the comfort and companionship of their twin. The joy that they inspire simply by being together and by starting to interact with each other is immeasurable. Whether they will grow up as best friends or sworn enemies remains to be seen, but theirs is a unique relationship that most parents hope they can help their children to nurture and cherish.

Parents of twins need to come to terms with the fact that they can't split themselves in half and therefore their way of doing things will be different – but no less effective – to parents who only have one baby.

Perfect parenting and other myths

Most people have a picture in their head of the sort of parent they hope to be. It may involve images of fun, playful times in a sunny park, making the babies giggle in the bath or cuddling together as you read a bedtime story. Or perhaps your babies will sit adorably in their high chairs as you enjoy a relaxed Sunday lunch with family and friends.

It almost certainly doesn't include sitting in your dressing gown at 2 p.m. picking half-chewed pieces of rice cake from your hair while offering a silent prayer that your grizzling babies will finally succumb to their afternoon nap. Or pacing up and down the living room in the small hours, wondering why your tiny baby will not stop crying.

The chances are, you'll have your fair share of both sides of the parenting coin, but there will be plenty of days when you feel you've had far more silent prayers than giggles. It can feel like you are stuck on the hard shoulder while everyone around you roars down the motorway of family life. No one has an easy time with a new baby, especially two new babies, including that glamourous woman in the cafe who looks to be breezing through motherhood. If you have other children, too, then you need to be realistic about what the fun–hard work ratio is likely to be.

66 From the moment your twins are born you'll become: athlete, chef, chemist, cleaner, clothes chooser, doctor, entertainer, gymnast, laundry manager, maker of toys, master multitasker, nurse, photographer, professional baby bather, psychologist, social organiser (for them, for you not so much), washer-upper and weightlifter (they get heavy!) 99

Kaz, mum to Nathaniel and Reuben, five

66 Your mantra should be: 'I am the best mother/father these babies have,' because you are! 99

Dr Bonamy Oliver, developmental psychologist with special expertise in twin families

66 What is important for the first year is feeding, clothing, setting routines and not being too stressed. It is about survival and being good enough. 99

Dr Sarah Helps, consultant clinical psychologist and family therapist, and mum to 12-year-old twins

66 I was so lucky to have a wonderful health visitor who kept drumming into me in the early weeks that you don't have to be perfect and that what you should be is good enough. Most twin mums beat themselves up with what they are missing – the cuddles, the time, the attention. Just as you feel you are having a special moment you have to put him down and tend to the other one. Just because they are not getting what singletons have doesn't mean they don't have other things – namely their relationship, which is a precious, magical thing. 99

Meryl, mum to Harri and Gethin, seven

When you are caring for twins who generally want or need the same things at the same time, it is easy to see them as a unit rather than two quite different people. One of the skills a parent of twins has to learn is how to make the time in an already busy day to forge individual relationships with their babies. If you have other children, too, as discussed in Chapter 6, then encouraging siblings to develop their own independent relationships is also important.

Tips for encouraging independence and taking turns:

▶ Sharing is great, and sometimes twins are good at it, but being forced to share doesn't work. If in doubt, ask yourself how you would feel if someone took your favourite book/CD/item of clothing/last bit of chocolate, and gave it to someone else and said, 'It's nice to share'!

▶ If you set up patterns of taking turns early, with luck, your babies will grow up accepting this, which may make one-on-one time easier as they get older. Even when they are really little, you can explain that it is 'Sasha's turn' to read a book and then 'Ella's turn'.

▶ Try to have a daily ten-minute play with each baby, focusing on one baby at a time. Explain that it is 'Ella's special time' and then 'Sasha's special time'. Alternate which baby goes first to keep things fair.

▶ Make sure that each baby has some of their own toys, which can be kept in their own box or area.

As well as keeping track of each baby's food intake, sleep patterns and nappy changes, parents of twins are also juggling a mental spreadsheet of how many kisses and cuddles each baby has received, and are doing their best to keep the score more or less even. Illness and crankiness can skew the balance a little, and sometimes a more demanding baby learns that this is a great way of getting extra attention from Mummy or Daddy.

All children have to endure a certain amount of comparison with their siblings, but with twins this can develop into an unhelpful shorthand for telling them apart. One twin may be known as 'the noisy one' or 'the shy one' – a label that may stick even if it is no longer the case, and maybe never was. Over the next few years, they will probably take it in turns to be 'noisy' or 'good' or 'confident' or 'cheeky', as well as many other things, just like any other child.

> ❝ Right from the beginning – from how they latch on, or sleep, or cry – parents start to tell themselves stories about their children, which can take on a life of their own. These stories about the character of their children start to shape the character of the child. You start to talk about the fussy child or the grumpy child or the smiley child. Sometimes these stories are helpful but sometimes children can start to act into the more negative ways in which they are described. It can be helpful to reflect on these stories and consider whether they are helpful or unhelpful, as you might find that the stories or descriptions only capture part of the child's character and skill. One way of taking a step back is to watch home videos of your children and really look at how you and others are interacting with each other. We all miss the positive things that our children do; try to hold on to these as you describe your children to others or when talking to the children themselves. ❞
>
> *Dr Sarah Helps, consultant clinical psychologist and family therapist, and mum to 12-year-old twins*

> ❝ I saw them too much as a unit. I found myself referring to the girls as 'they' a lot and lumping them together, even though they were actually quite different from pretty early on. You have to see them as two individual children. ❞
>
> *Mandie, mum to Lara and Zadie, two; and Rhys, four*

Parents often feel the only way they can be seen to treat their twins fairly is to give them the same things at the same time, but often this isn't necessary and can set you up for some murderously expensive shopping trips. It is also another barrier to seeing your children as individuals, if you treat them the same regardless of what each person actually needs. Your children need to be confident that they will be treated fairly but they also need to be aware that this won't always mean they get the same thing.

> ❝ Treating your twins identically is not necessarily helpful for the children. It also won't necessarily avoid the arguments! Children need to be treated fairly, but that's not the same as identically. Help them to understand that fairness isn't always getting the same thing at the same time – their needs can be different. For example, if only one child needs shoes, you won't get them both shoes.
>
> If one child is being disruptive it is tempting to spend more time dealing with that, rather than being with the child who is behaving calmly, but fairness is also about making sure that the 'easier' child receives the same amount of acknowledgement and attention when you can.

Sometimes you can take it as a useful chance to show both children behaviours that you'd like to see. For example, if Franky is yelling and bashing bricks together, and Billy is sitting calmly playing, without saying anything to Franky, you can say, 'You're playing nicely, Billy.' Don't use this as a moment to compare, or say anything negative to Franky, but instead simply as a moment to praise Billy: that way, the message to both children is that this is the behaviour that gets attention. 99

Dr Bonamy Oliver, developmental psychologist with special expertise in twin families

See Chapter 9 for more parenting techniques for twins.

The twin bond

Most parents of twins are not twins themselves and are as fascinated about the twin relationship as everyone else. However, as discussed in Chapter 20, not all twins grow up to become best friends and, disappointingly, very few develop telepathic powers. In short, your twins will always be twins but, in common with all siblings, their relationships will vary tremendously. Some twins can't wait to break free of the 'twin' tag, while others love the extra dimension and security that they feel their relationship gives them.

66 People can worry about whether the twin bond is special, whether it should be special, or whether it's weird, or whether they'll argue or be best friends. But actually they are just two people.

It is important to acknowledge the twins' relationship, because it is part of who they are. But it is also important to allow that relationship to develop as they want it to develop. Most parents don't know what it's like to be a twin and sometimes their ideas are not based in reality. Show the children about love and kindness generally and nurture the relationship from afar, try not to artificially create something between them – let it develop as your twins want it to. "

Dr Bonamy Oliver, developmental psychologist with special expertise in twin families

All parents tie themselves up in knots, worrying that the choices they make in good faith will in some way backfire or be held up in 20 years' time as the reason behind underachievement or lack of confidence in their children. Parenting twins is an extra, happy twist in an already complicated world.

No one knows what sort of adults your twins will become, but with the gift of unconditional love, encouragement and the knowledge that they are cherished individuals, their future is surely bright.

Chapter 20

Being a Twin

It seems only right that it should be twins themselves who have the final word in this book, because although the dreaded question 'What's it like, being a twin?' will drive your children to distraction, it is probably exactly what we're all secretly wondering.

As these adult twins demonstrate perfectly, it is a question to which there are as many answers as there are twins. Your twins, like all others, will brave the flashbulbs and curiosity, and emerge into adulthood with a unique relationship, not as others expect it to be, but as they want it to be. It will be a blast and a privilege to be along for the ride.

My twin and I...

“ My first memory is of us starting school. They wanted to separate us and we stood in the hallway holding on to each other, sobbing. As a child I felt like I had one up on my other friends. I couldn't imagine what it must be like to grow up a single child. Being a twin is really wonderful and is so special. Christina is my partner for life, not by choice, but by a wonderful twist of fate.

Christina and I once both had a crush on the same guy and he chose Christina. Strangely, I don't remember feeling bad about that – he made his choice and obviously I was disappointed, but I didn't feel we were in competition.

I think the only negative side effect of being a twin is guilt. Every decision that I made, especially in my teens and early

263

20s, I would ask myself how Christina was going to feel about it. You've got your partner in life but you need to find another partner, too, and we certainly found that the initial stages of forming a long-term relationship were quite wobbly. You have to give up some physical proximity if you want to get more from life and that can be hard. 99

Natalie, 31, twin of Christina; and sister of Daniel, 27

66 When I meet new people and tell them I'm a twin they always assume my sister must be my best friend and she isn't — we're not even that close. We get on when we see each other, but we aren't really close.

My parents were brilliant, but I wish other people had treated us as individuals — sometimes it felt like we were the same person. There are so many more things about us than the fact that we are twins.

When we were younger I used the twin thing almost as a shield. I was very shy and Lucy was more confident, and I'd expect her to do things first. With hindsight, that probably didn't do much for my self-esteem.

Lucy is amazing at art and I had the same teacher as her. He would always come over to me and suggest things, based on what my sister had done on her work. He called me 'the rebel', while Lucy was the amazing artist. I don't think I was particularly rebellious — I just didn't like art.

As a teenager I really wanted to look different from Lucy. I cut my hair and dyed it, while she had long brown hair, and really tried to make my own identity.

One thing that still sticks in my mind even though it happened so many years ago, is when a great aunt phoned. I answered and she said: 'Are you the arty one or are you the other one?'

We've both got really bad self-esteem and I do think it is because we're twins. We've always had someone else to compare ourselves against. I still do it — I look at her life and wonder if it's better than mine or if that is what I should be doing, whereas I never think that about my brother. 🙄

Emily, 22, identical twin of Lucy; and sister of Charlie, 18

💬 Tom was always much brighter than me, always way ahead, but I never resented it, or even thought about it. I was pony-obsessed and nothing else really came into it!

Tom went off to do national service. I never knew what happened to him, but when he came back he had a massive nervous breakdown and I was the only one allowed to know, he wouldn't tell my parents.

As adults we always had this kind of telepathy between us – if something bad or difficult was happening to the other one, we'd get a sense that something was wrong which would usually be confirmed with a phone call or letter. One time I was living in Zambia and was engaged to Peter (who I've now been married to for 44 years). Peter had been married before and suddenly had cold feet about whether he wanted to do it again and for a short time it wasn't certain whether the engagement would continue. Almost the same day I got a letter from Tom which said, 'Something is troubling you. I hope all is well with you and Peter'. This happened fairly frequently and we were always right.

Tom had quite poor mental health for most of his life and I hope I was always there for him. He was a great letter writer, even though his handwriting was terrible and an absolute agony to read. He would send me these long letters, sometimes full of optimism and reminiscences about our childhood, other times they were low and he was at rock bottom. He died three years ago, and I have become estranged from his daughter, which is something I never imagined could happen. She is my only link to my twin brother now, and it seems very sad to have lost that. 🙄

Mary, 79, twin of Tom, who died aged 76

66 My sister and I have always been close and have always done things together. We were in the same class in junior school and then had different tutors at secondary school, but still saw each other. Midway through, when I was about 13, I had to go to a different school and I remember crying because I didn't want to be away from Riah.

I've always talked to her and trusted her, and her opinion means more to me than anyone else's. That said, my mum hates being in the same room as us sometimes because we take the micky and give each other abuse, but it's all just joking around.

We have twin brothers who are three years older but they are not close at all – there has always been rivalry and they don't really speak much. I don't think there's anything you can do to make twins close or best friends – it either happens or it doesn't. 99

Leon, 31, twin of Riah; and brother of twins Dominic and Richard, 34

66 Samantha and I were close as young children and played together a lot. Our parents divorced when we were seven. We moved with mum to a new home in a new town and everything changed. Even the dog, who we'd had since it was a puppy was given away. Without wanting to sound dramatic, we were a broken family.

As primary school progressed, we found our own friends and spent less time together. After the divorce my mum enrolled me in the Navy Training Corps, which is a bit like the Sea Cadets, and after a bit my mum and sister joined, too. It meant that we used to do a lot together – we were in the band and at the weekends would be off canoeing, which was great, but when we reached the age that we'd rather be doing other things and left, family life started to fragment a bit.

My sister and I went to different secondary schools – she went to the state girls' school and I went to the boys' school, which was just down the road. For a 13-year-old boy, the fact that I had a sister at the girls' school was fantastic!

Mum and my sister used to fight quite a bit as Samantha was going through the teenage years and by comparison I was seen as the blue-eyed boy who could do no wrong. My sister got into quite a lot of trouble and didn't do well at school. The last straw was when my mum caught her in town when she should have been at work, and she was sent to live with my dad and his new family. My dad then decided that they were all going to live in Florida! So, the 'punishment' for my sister for being kicked out of home was to go to Florida for a few years and as a 16-year-old boy stuck at home I felt really hard done by.

We hardly spoke to each other for years after that. She phoned me on our 18th birthday, but we didn't get back together until we were 21. She was back from the States and had her first child not long after. Since then we've probably only seen each other on average about once a year, and there have been periods lasting years when I haven't heard a word from her. We have tended to hear about each other through our parents.

Now I am married and have two young sons, and obviously you think about your childhood and it influences the way you are as a parent. For us, the communication wasn't there – there was a lot of resentment on both sides, but never once have we spoken about it. Now with my sons I hope they will talk to me if they have problems.

I think my mum is a bit gutted that we aren't close, and recently she's been trying to get us together a bit more. At the moment, she wants us all to go on holiday together next year, which I have agreed to. Sometimes you've got to take one for the team, and this is for my mum.

My oldest son and Samantha's son adore each other and talk about each other all the time, so there is a link there. Despite the negative things I've said, my sister is a really caring person and has a heart of gold. She is training to be a nurse now, which she will be really good at. She has held out the olive branch recently. We'll see how the holiday goes. 🗩

Matt, 41, twin of Samantha

🗨 We were a family of 11 children, including three sets of twins, which even with the big families of that time was unusual. At one point Mammy had six kids under five – I don't know how she did it. She only died last year, aged 99 and half, so it can't have been so bad!

There was a bond between all the twins except for me and Maureen. According to my parents, she was born half an hour before me and was always to be called their eldest daughter. This was fine with me, as she was the one expected to do all the work.

Maureen was exceptionally clever and it was decided that she wouldn't get a proper education in Ireland so she and I were sent to my daddy's sister, our Auntie Maureen, who lived near Manchester and didn't have any children. We got there in time to take our 11-plus, which I failed and Maureen passed, so she went to a good convent school as planned and I went to the secondary modern. However, she absolutely hated the whole set-up and within six months had run away. Daddy had to come over and get her, but I felt sorry for my auntie so I stayed. I liked being an only child and stayed until I was 14.

Maureen said she was never going to use her brain, she was going to get married and have a lot of kids and that's what she did. She had seven children, including a set of twins, and never left Ireland again. I felt differently, though, and left Ireland for England when I was 19. When I arrived in Liverpool it felt like I'd come home. I go back to Ireland, but I have never wanted to live there again. I have probably seen Maureen every two or three years since then. I don't think our twin bond is especially close, I am closer to one of my other sisters than Maureen.

I have three children, two boys and a girl, but no twins. I would have liked my daughter to be twins – I'd have liked twin girls. 99

Ann, 73, twin of Maureen; and sister to Paul, 76; Sean and Seamus, 75; Cathleen, 71; Roseleen, 70; Charlie, 66; Gerry and Bernadette, 62; Noelle (who died in her 20s); and Dennis, 61

66 I've always had a really close bond with Andy. One of my warmest memories is sitting in the bath together eating Rice Krispies. When we were little kids I remember him biting and bullying me and having to hide under the television stand, but then the next minute we were having great fights with potato guns – leaving my mum to clear up the mess, I'm sure. We've never been competitive and have stayed close, although there have been difficult patches in both our lives when we've gone our own ways and found our own path out of it. We don't live in each other's pockets but he would always be the first person I'd call if I needed help, and I hope I'd be the first person he'd call. As much as I love my sisters, Andy is my first love and I can't think of anything he could do to break that. 99

Stewart, 53, twin of Andrew; and brother of Susan, Jane and Jill

66 We were born by emergency C-section only a few weeks after Mum discovered she was expecting twins and they didn't find out if there was one placenta or two. The one question everyone wants to know is if you are identical and we didn't know, but as we got older our curiosity grew. When we were 18 we decided to find out ourselves and the

DNA test came back that we were a 99.9 per cent match. I remember feeling that it was a relief to finally have an answer to the question that had always hung over us.

My husband is a twin, too – our mothers met in confinement in hospital and knitted together while they waited for us to arrive. We stayed in touch as families so Kit was always a feature in our life. Rachel was away travelling when Kit and I got together and I think she found it very difficult when he proposed and we became engaged. She was single at the time and we were all on holiday in France with Mum and Dad when Kit did the old-fashioned thing and asked my dad if he could marry me. We then went back to England and Mum told me that Rachel cried all the time. She knows I know she was upset, but I don't think we talked about it. She was great about the wedding though and helped me with it and was a bridesmaid. Her husband, Spencer, and mine get on really well, although I think Spencer still finds it a bit weird that he's married to an identical twin. Both our husbands are very supportive of us spending time with each other and are not threatened by the closeness of our relationship. We're not weird about it, but we talk quite often on the phone, and we see each other every few months.

Rachel and I have always been emotionally very robust but that may be because we've got each other. Our older and younger sisters are both quite anxious and highly strung, and it might be that mine and Rachel's relationship has informed that.

The thing that makes our relationship different from any other is knowing that she understands me and I totally understand her. I can be totally honest and straightforward about things. There is an implicit understanding that whatever you say is OK. She hears when I talk and just gets why I do things – I don't need to explain. I feel totally safe in her presence or the knowledge of her presence. 〞

Louise, 38, twin of Rachel; sister of Kate, 40, and Alice, 28

Resources and Further Reading

Resources

Twin parenting information and support

▶ Multiple Births Foundation – A charity dedicated to offering advice, expertise and support for parents of twins, triplets and quads – www.multiplebirths.org.uk

▶ Twins and Multiple Births Association (TAMBA) – Lots of advice, including a helpline and forum. You can get discounts at certain shops if you become a member – www.tamba.org.uk

▶ Twins UK – An online support resource that also sells twin-related items – www.twinsuk.co.uk

Twins clubs

Find your nearest club via TAMBA or Twins UK (see above). Your local authority should also be able to recommend any local twins playgroups.

Infertility support

Infertility Network UK – www.infertilitynetworkuk.com

Healthy eating during pregnancy

▶ British Dietetic Association pregnancy food facts – www.bda.uk.com/foodfacts/Pregnancy.pdf

▶ 'Optimal Nutrition for Improved Twin Pregnancy Outcome' by William Goodnight and Roger Newman for the Society of

Maternal-Fetal Medicine, published by American College of Obstetricians and Gynecologists

- 'The Healthy Multiple Pregnancy Guide' by Dr Erika McAslan Fraser, published by TAMBA

- NHS Healthy Start – Healthy eating advice and details of a scheme providing vouchers for milk, fruit and vegetables – www.healthystart.nhs.uk

Maternity leave and your rights
Maternity Action – www.maternityaction.org.uk

Twin-to-twin transfusion syndrome support
- 'Twin-to-Twin Transfusion Syndrome: A Guide for Parents' by Dr Erika McAslan Fraser, published by TAMBA

- Twin to Twin Transfusion Syndrome UK parents – Closed Facebook support group for UK parents facing this condition – www.facebook.com/groups/324913884215990

Premature birth
- Bliss – A charity which supports parents and their premature babies as well as campaigning on their behalf for the best possible care and support – www.bliss.org.uk

- Tommy's – A charity which funds research into the causes of premature birth, stillbirth and miscarriage – www.tommys.org

Birth
- Birth Choice UK – A detailed analysis of maternity facilities across the UK – www.birthchoiceuk.com

- Birth Trauma Association – A support group for women who have had a traumatic birth experience – www.birthtraumaassociation.org.uk

▶ National Institute for Health and Care Excellence (NICE) – For information on national clinical guidelines for multiple births – www.nice.org.uk

▶ Royal College of Obstetricians and Gynaecologists – For information on the profession's multiple birth guidelines – www.rcog.org.uk

Breastfeeding support

▶ Association of Breastfeeding Mothers – A breastfeeding support organisation which offers a helpline and online chats – abm.me.uk

▶ La Leche League GB – Breastfeeding support – www.laleche.org.uk

▶ The Breastfeeding Network – Help, support and independent information about breastfeeding – www.breastfeedingnetwork.org.uk

Sleep support

▶ Cry-Sis – Support for families with excessively crying, sleepless or demanding babies – www.cry-sis.org.uk

▶ Lullaby Trust – Expert advice on safer baby sleep and special support for anyone bereaved through sudden infant death syndrome (SIDS) – www.lullabytrust.org.uk

Home safety

▶ Child Accident Prevention Trust – A charity that works to reduce the number of children and young people killed, disabled or seriously injured in accidents – www.capt.org.uk

Help at home

▶ Doula UK – An organisation which provides parents with information about doulas as well as offering guidance and support to doulas themselves – www.doula.org.uk

- Doula UK Access Fund – Information on how to access a doula if your household income is less than £16,000 a year – www.doula.org.uk/doula-access-fund

- Family and Childcare Trust – An organisation which supports family life, with lots of information and research about childcare – www.familyandchildcaretrust.org

- Home-Start – A charity which provides volunteers to help and support families in their own homes – www.home-start.org.uk

- Independent Midwives UK – A membership organisation for independent midwives which offers advice about how to find your local independent midwife – www.imuk.org.uk

Postnatal depression

- Mind – Offers advice and support on all aspects of mental health – www.mind.org.uk

- Pandas – Advice on both pre and postnatal depression – www.pandasfoundation.org.uk

- 'Postnatal Depression: A Guide for Mothers of Multiples' by Dr Erika McAslan Fraser, published by TAMBA

Communication

- Talking Point – A website about children's speech, language and communication, designed for parents and people who work with children – www.talkingpoint.org.uk

- The Communication Trust – A coalition of organisations which support people who work with children to support their speech, language and communication. Contains useful links to early years communication resources – www.thecommunicationtrust.org.uk

▶ National Literacy Trust – Tools for parents to help their children develop communication and literacy skills from birth – www.literacytrust.org.uk

Relationships

▶ Relate – Offers counselling for every type of relationship – www.relate.org.uk

▶ The Couple Connection – A forum with information and advice about relationships – www.thecoupleconnection.net

LGBT

We Are Family – LGBT parenting magazine – www.wearefamilymagazine.co.uk

Single parents

Gingerbread – A charity which offers support and advice for single parents – www.gingerbread.org.uk

Domestic violence

▶ National Domestic Violence Helpline 0808 2000 247 (24 hours)

▶ Refuge – Help for women and children who have suffered as a result of domestic abuse – www.refuge.org.uk

Further reading

Books on raising twins

▶ *Double Trouble* by Emma Mahony (Thorsons, 2003)

▶ *Ready or Not... Here We Come!* by Elizabeth Lyons (Finn-Phyllis Press, 2007)

▶ *Twins and the Family* by Audrey Sandbank (Arrow Books, 1988)

▶ *We Are Twins, But Who Am I?* by Betty Jean Case (Tibbut Publishers, 1991)

Books preparing siblings for the arrival of twins

▶ *I'm Having Twins!* by Paris Morris (New Year Publishing, 2008)

▶ *My Mum's Going to Explode!* by Jeremy Strong (Puffin, 2007)

▶ *Princess Poppy: The Baby Twins* by Janey Louise Jones (Picture Corgi, 2007)

Young children's books featuring twins

▶ *Bathtime for Twins* by Ellen Weiss (Little Simon, 2012)

▶ *Chimp and Zee* series by Catherine and Laurence Anholt

▶ *Just Like Me* by Barbara Neasi and Johanna Hantel (Scholastic, 2011)

▶ *My Name is Ellie* by Meran R. Robinson (Amazon, 2015)

▶ *Rip and Rap* by Amanda White (Barefoot Books Ltd, 2003)

▶ *Topsy and Tim* series by Jean and Gareth Adamson

▶ *Two is for Twins* by Wendy Cheyette Lewison (Viking, 2011)

Books about routine

▶ *A Contented House with Twins* by Gina Ford and Alice Beer (Vermillion, 2006)

▶ *Baby Secrets: How to Know Your Baby's Needs* by Jo Tantum and Barbara Want (a mother of twins) (Michael Joseph, 2005)

▶ *The Baby Sleep Guide* by Stephanie Modell (a mother of triplets) (Vie, 2015)

▶ *The Baby Whisperer* by Tracy Hogg (Vermillion, 2005)

Credits

pp.157–158: World Health Organization guidelines on bottle feeding reprinted from *How to Prepare Formula for Bottle-feeding at Home*, published by the Department of Food Safety, Zoonoses and Foodborne Diseases, WHO, in collaboration with the Food and Agriculture Organization of the United Nations (FAO), pp.4–5, 2008.

p.228: Information on communication reproduced courtesy of The National Literacy Trust.

About the Author

Jessica Bomford is a journalist, writer and nagger-in-chief to her three sons. Her life changed course when her second baby turned out to be identical twins and has remained on an uneven keel ever since. She is married and lives in London.

If you would like to tell Jessica about your twins or have any comments about the book, join the It's Twins! Now What? community at **www.facebook.com/twinsnowwhat**.

Glossary

anaesthetist – A doctor who specialises in pain relief and anaesthesia

antenatal – Before birth

baby-led weaning (BLW) – A method of weaning that allows babies to feed themselves on suitable solid 'first foods'

Braxton Hicks contractions – Painless contractions of the uterus that can be experienced throughout pregnancy

caesarean/C-section – A surgical method of delivering babies by cutting through the abdomen and then into the womb (uterus)

catheter (urinary) – When a tube is inserted into the body to drain and collect urine from the bladder

colic – A term used for excessive, frequent crying in a baby who appears to be otherwise healthy which begins at a few weeks old and normally stops by four to six months

colostrum – First breast milk, a nutrient-dense thick, yellow liquid which also contains antibodies and white blood cells to protect babies from infection

cry it out – A sleep-training method which allows a baby to cry for a specified, usually short, period of time before offering comfort

developmental hip dysplasia – When the ball and socket of the hip joint do not fit snugly together, resulting in varying degrees of severity

dizygotic – Twins which result from two separate eggs, released at the same ovulation time, which were fertilised by two different sperm. The twins will be 'non-identical'

epidural – Where painkillers are passed to the small of your back via a fine tube

flat head syndrome/plagiocephaly – A condition characterised by a flattening on one side of the back of the head. It may also involve bulging of the forehead, fullness of the cheek and ear misalignment on the same side as the flattening

fontanelle – Two soft spots on the top of a newborn baby's head (a diamond shaped patch near the front and a smaller spot towards the back) where the skull bone has not yet fused together

gas and air – A mixture of oxygen and nitrous oxide gas offered as a first pain relief to women in labour

gestational diabetes – During pregnancy, some women have such high levels of blood glucose that their body is unable to produce enough insulin to absorb it all, this is known as gestational diabetes. It disappears after the baby is born

GP – A general practitioner; a doctor who works from a local practice

gradual retreat – A sleep-training method which allows parents to gradually retreat from their crying babies, starting with patting, to sitting by the cot, to, eventually, leaving the room altogether

health visitor – Specially trained nurses who support families from pregnancy to the child's fifth birthday, if required

hypnobirthing – An approach to birth which involves self-hypnosis, relaxation and breathing techniques

ICSI – Intracytoplasmic sperm injection is a technique in which a single sperm is injected into the centre of an egg and is the favoured fertilisation method for all types of IVF

intrauterine growth restriction (IGR) – When one or both unborn babies are smaller than expected, which can lead to problems for the baby/ies or result in an early delivery

in utero – Latin term meaning 'in the womb'

in-vitro fertilisation (IVF) – This is the original 'test-tube' baby technique where a woman's eggs are collected and then fertilised in a test tube to create several embryos which are transferred to the uterus, where, hopefully, they implant and a pregnancy begins

mastitis – When a woman's breast tissue becomes painful and inflamed, often caused by a build-up of milk within the breast

midwife – An expert in normal pregnancy and birth, some have particular expertise in multiple births

monozygotic – Twins that result from one fertilised egg, which splits very early in pregnancy. The twins will be 'identical'

NCT – National Childbirth Trust, a charity for parents

neonatal – Provision of care for newborn babies

NICU – Neonatal intensive care unit

obstetrician – A doctor who specialises in the care of women during pregnancy, labour and birth

oxytocin – Often called the 'love hormone' which has many effects, including helping to bring on contractions and promoting the 'let down' reflex, which allows breast milk to come through

paediatrician – A doctor who specialises in the care of babies and children

perineum – The area between the anus and the vagina

pessary – A medical device inserted into the vagina to administer medication

placenta praevia – When a placenta is lying low in the uterus, blocking or partially blocking the babies' exits

postnatal – After birth

postnatal depression (PND) – Depression brought on by a number of factors following birth, but can develop at any time during the first year after birth

pre-eclampsia – A type of high blood pressure that only happens in pregnancy and can cause complications for both mothers and their babies

prem/preemie – Premature baby, i.e. born before 37 weeks

ranitidine – A prescription drug used, in some cases, to treat reflux

respiratory syncytial virus (RSV) – A common virus that may cause a cough or cold, but in young children can trigger more serious infections of the lungs and respiratory tract

runner – Support staff in the operating theatre. They may transfer patients between the wards and the operating theatre or look after equipment in theatre, and ensure the area stays clean and tidy

sciatica – This is the name given to any sort of pain that is caused by irritation or compression of the sciatic nerve, which runs from the back of the pelvis, through the buttocks, and all the way down both legs, ending at the feet

scrub nurse – Specialist nurses who care for patients in a surgical environment (i.e. the operating theatre)

sonographer – Someone specially trained to carry out ultrasound scans

spina bifida – A permanently disabling birth defect, literally meaning 'split spine', when the spinal column does not close all of the way, which happens when the baby is in the womb

sudden infant death syndrome – Formerly known as 'cot death', this is an unexplained, unexpected and sudden death of an apparently healthy baby. About 300 babies a year die from this

supervisor of midwives – An experienced midwife who can support and help you if you are having problems with your care or feel your wishes are not being considered

Syntocinon – A brand name for oxytocin (see above), which may be administered in hospital to speed up labour

twin-to-twin transfusion syndrome – When twins share a placenta there can be an uneven bloodflow between the foetuses, resulting in one twin having too much supply, resulting in a strain on the heart as it works harder to cope, and the other gets too little blood, which affects its growth

vanishing twin syndrome (VTS) – A pregnancy which begins as twins, but one embryo fails to thrive and is absorbed into the womb thus 'disappearing' by the 12-week scan

vernix – Waxy white substance found coating the skin of newborn babies

zygote – One fertilised egg

Index

Have you enjoyed this book?
If so, why not write a review on your favourite website?

If you're interested in finding out more about our books,
find us on Facebook at **Summersdale Publishers** and follow us
on Twitter at **@Summersdale**.

Thanks very much for buying this Summersdale book.

www.summersdale.com